WITHDRAWN FROM STOCK

# EXERCISE THROUGHOUT LIFE

## Also by Peter F. Williams

Adventure Training/Recreational
*Canoeing Skills and Canoe Expedition Techniques for Teachers and Leaders*
(Pelham)
*Camping and Hill Trekking* (Pelham)
*Beginners' Guide to Lightweight Camping* (Pelham)
*Camping Complete* (Pelham)
*Canoeing* (Pelham)
*Hill Walking* (Pelham)
*Adventure Camping* (Pelham)

Fiction (written under the pseudonym Peter Wellesbourne)
*Operation Albatross* (Robert Hale)
*Bomb New York* (Robert Hale)

# EXERCISE
## THROUGHOUT LIFE

**PETER F. WILLIAMS**

MAINSTREAM
PUBLISHING

EDINBURGH AND LONDON

*Exercise throughout Life* is dedicated to my wife Glenys, at one time all-weather rugby supporter, kayak carrier, tent erector, Wahiba Sands desert driver, accomplished secretary and supportive Service wife in peace and war. My Inspiration.

First published in Great Britain in 2000 by
MAINSTREAM PUBLISHING COMPANY (EDINBURGH) LTD
7 Albany Street
Edinburgh EH1 3UG

ISBN 1 84018 273 3

A catalogue record for this book is available from the British Library

Typeset in Gill Sans and Stone Serif
Printed and bound in Great Britain by Creative Print Design, Wales

# Contents

# Illustrations, Tests and Programmes

# Acknowledgements

The author wishes to record his appreciation of the helpful comments received on the draft of this book from the following:

Dr Angela Fairney, MD, FRCP, FRCPath, Lead Consultant, Osteoporosis Clinic, St Mary's NHS Trust and Imperial College School of Medicine, London; Gp Capt P.L. Watson, DPhysEd, FIMgt, MBISA, RAF, Director of Physical Education RAF; Wg Cdr P. Rooney, BA, DPhysEd, MBIFM, RAF, Officer Commanding, the RAF School of Physical Training, RAF Cosford; Dr Olga Rutherford, BA, MSc, PhD, Lecturer in Physiology, Imperial College of Medicine, London; Wayne M. Thomas, MPhil, formerly Llanelli RFC; Dr Judith Hall, MB, BS, LRCP, MRCS, Osteoporosis Clinic, St Mary's NHS Trust, London; and Dr Robert Lambert, BSc, PhD, CChem, FRSC, formerly London University RFC.

The author is also indebted to the Health Education Authority for permission to publish extracts from their booklet, *Exercise – Why Bother?*

# The Chance of Your Lifetime

- The Benefits of Exercise
- The Human Body
- Exercise through Life
- Meeting Challenges with Fitness

How active are you? Why do I ask? Your life could depend upon it. Each year coronary heart disease (CHD) kills about 150,000 people in the United Kingdom. What causes CHD?

Unlike some diseases, such as tuberculosis or asbestosis, CHD does not have a single cause but is a condition related to a number of risk factors. Some, such as genetic background, race, or increased age, cannot be changed. However, there are other risk factors that are within your control. These are cigarette smoking, excessive calorie intake, raised cholesterol levels, high alcohol intake, degree of stress and lack of physical exercise. When more than one of these factors is present the risk of dying from coronary heart disease increases considerably. There are other diseases and disorders that can affect the quality of our lives. Osteoporosis (a disorder of the bones) and osteoporotic fractures have, according to some experts, become an epidemic in the industrialised world and as a result of modern lifestyle our children could, in years to come as they grow into adulthood, be at risk. So what can you do? I'll tell you.

It is believed that adequate amounts of physical activity carried out regularly can improve health and prevent disease. A working party of the Royal College of Physicians concluded that there is good evidence of the many physical and psychological benefits available to the population from regular exercise.[1] So when is exercise best started? The Royal College of Physicians recommends that the habit of taking regular recreational exercise is best started in childhood; should be continued into middle age; and taken where possible into old age, because exercise helps to make the most of diminishing physical capacity. *Exercise throughout Life* aims to encourage people of all ages, from childhood to beyond retirement, to participate in regular exercise of their choice, so establishing an exercise pattern and developing a sound standard of physical fitness and a healthy lifestyle.

Over the last decade there has been a steady increase in the number of people, young and older, who are interested in being active and keeping fit. Some people become involved in aerobic classes, fitness clubs or weight training; some take up sports or games. There are many who seek to maintain or improve their level of physical fitness through a form of interesting personal exercise programme, but may not have the guidance on what form of exercise is possible and how to select, then start, a suitable programme. This book offers that guidance. For other people the end of school can mean the end of any opportunity, however limited, of taking part in sport and physical exercise. Work undertaken often involves very little physical exertion unless a manual occupation is pursued. The too frequent use of the motor car, and other trends of modern life, tend to lead to a sedentary lifestyle. People may drive too much and walk too little. By the time they are in their late 20s or even earlier, may have given up sport or other forms of strenuous activity. However, it is never too late to take part in exercise, for the benefits of doing so are well proven and considerable.

THE BENEFITS OF EXERCISE

There are many very good reasons why regular exercise should be an ongoing pattern of our lifestyle and they apply to young and old alike. Some are physical, mental and social and are

[1] P.H. Fentem, 'ABC of Sports Medicine', *British Medical Journal*, vol. 308, 14 May 1994.

summarised by the Health Education Authority and Sports Council as follows:

a. Exercise helps you feel good in mind and body.
b. It's great fun and a good way of making new friends and enjoying your leisure time more.
c. It helps you feel more energetic.
d. It helps you relax.
e. It helps you get slim and stay slim.
f. It helps keep you supple and more mobile as you get older.
g. It helps strengthen your muscles, joints and even your bones.
h. It improves the staying power of your muscles.
i. It helps your heart work more efficiently, improves your circulation and helps protect against heart disease.
j. It helps almost everything in your body work better.
k. It needn't cost anything.
l. And it gets easier the more you do.[1]

Regular exercise also helps prevent the onset of types of diabetes, reduces the risk of cancer of the colon and lowers blood cholesterol levels.

THE HUMAN BODY

The human body is a unique and fine machine but it is one of the few machines that will degenerate and break down if not used. The longer the inactivity, the greater the possibility of a malfunction in one or several of the body's complex systems, whether the systems relate to heart, circulation, respiration or joints. Our body therefore needs to be used regularly and properly so that its systems are kept in good shape.

In addition there is one significant reason why regular exercise should be taken throughout our lives. Regular exercise promotes bone formation, growth and strength in the important period of body development – from childhood to well into the 20s – and is therefore essential to the

[1] Reproduced with the permission of the Health Education Authority.

development of a sound body. As you grow older it helps protect the bones from becoming brittle and more susceptible to bone fractures and the disability of osteoporosis (see chapter 3). This particular disorder may result in deformity and can be painful when bones become porous and break. It affects one in four women and one in twelve men. Medical studies have revealed that exercise has a very important part to play in the prevention and treatment of osteoporosis. For many, regular exercise is an investment in the quality of life, both now and in the future.

## EXERCISE THROUGH LIFE

Older people can take satisfaction from the fact that there are now more people living to a greater age than ever before. Medical care, sensible diet and good housing are all contributing factors that influence the modern lifespan. A century or so ago 'toes-up' time arrived around 40 years of age, even less. We in the Western world are fortunate, for most people have a fair chance of living out their natural biological lifespan. The result is that there are more people reaching the age of retirement. The likely further reduction in retirement age will mean that even more people could, in the future, be in a position to look forward to a long, healthy, enjoyable period of active leisure time, provided they take steps to achieve and maintain a sound standard of fitness.

The way you approach retirement and the more mature years will depend very much on your attitude of mind and could influence the quality of your life. Those in the middle years can either regard their life as being half over or half yet to be lived, for middle age should not be regarded as a prelude to decline.

Until fairly recently I was privileged to know a very old gentleman. He was A.J. Sylvester, who had been personal private secretary to Lloyd George, the Prime Minister of Great Britain during the First World War. A.J. was energetic with an indomitable spirit. At the age of 80-plus he became UK Latin American ballroom dancing champion and featured in the Guinness Book of Records. He was also still driving his sports car. Even when he was into his 90s, A.J. rose early each day to work at his typewriter and record his remarkable diaries that spanned back to and before the First World War. He often said to me, 'Peter, I have a life's work ahead of me and the days are not long enough.' Sadly he did not make 100 years, only 99 years and 11 months. I like to think that his slightly premature call was due to the requirement for an experienced private secretary in heaven! But whatever the reason, I do believe that all those years ago, when A.J. had celebrated his 50th birthday, he felt he had half of his life left, to be lived fully and energetically.

## MEETING CHALLENGES WITH FITNESS

Perhaps our lives are marked with milestones – schooling, sporting and academic achievements, courtship, marriage and children. Some may have been sad – bereavement, divorce, war. But they are all experiences that, in a direct or indirect way, enrich our lives, whichever way we look at them. The same can be said for the future with all those other milestones yet to be reached and life to be further enriched. Whatever the challenges that lie ahead, the benefits inherent in a sound standard of fitness will enhance the quality of our lives and those of our children and grandchildren.

This book is written to give a clear understanding of the benefits of exercise and how a sound standard of fitness can be achieved at all ages. It outlines the various forms of basic fitness training and gives guidance on how to follow a programme of your choice that may also help avoid the onset of CHD and osteoporosis. It offers you your chance of a lifetime!

# ONE

## What is Physical Fitness?

- Types of Fitness
- How Fit are You?
  - A Simple Fitness Test
- The Three Major Components of Fitness
  - Stamina
  - Strength
    - Static Strength
    - Dynamic Strength
    - Explosive Strength
  - Suppleness
- Additional Components of Fitness
  - Speed
  - Skill

The word 'fitness' tends to be wrongly associated with vigorous competitive sport and the performance of super athletes, rather than the ability of ordinary people who display various degrees of fitness according to their role in life and the influence of the environment in which they operate. Most people want to feel and look fit and to be healthy. They also want to lead a healthy lifestyle. Many think that they are as fit as they need to be, yet some can find digging the garden too hard, or going for brisk walks too taxing. What, then, is this quality called fitness? How does it vary and how does it apply to you?

Physical fitness is a quality that can only be measured in relation to a specific task. The word 'fitness', as applied to physical conditioning, is a somewhat confusing term because different sports and activities have different requirements. For example, the ability of a weight-lifter to lift a massive weight proves that he has the physical ability to lift that weight, but does not prove he has the capacity to walk, run or cycle a long distance. Again, the ability to perform 30 press-ups or 20 burpees proves the ability to do such a task, but alone has little relevance to 'overall' or 'endurance' fitness (which reflects the overall health and efficiency of the heart, lungs and general musculature).

Some people measure fitness by degrees of muscular development, as seen in the muscular fitness of the weight-lifter, or in the degree of skills required in a specific sport. Various activities require different components of fitness, as shown in the dynamic speed required by the sprinter; the suppleness of the dancer and gymnast; and the stamina of the marathon runner. However, all of these sports specialities require some of the components that are present in their sporting counterparts. The sprinter, for example, requires a certain degree of strength, as does a ballet dancer, who also needs endurance.

At one extreme of the fitness scale is the standard required by the highly trained sportsman, sometimes described as 'total' fitness and involving the possession of strength, stamina and suppleness plus speed and skill. At the lower end of the scale is the level of fitness that typifies a sedentary lifestyle possessed by the non-exerciser, sometimes described as 'passive' fitness. It enables people to get to work, sit behind their desks and mix socially; but it hardly provides them with sufficient stamina or strength to climb several flights of stairs, or run for a bus, without becoming out of breath or even exhausted. In the middle of these two extremes is that level of 'general' fitness that is sufficient for a person to cope with work and to carry out daily tasks, yet also provides sufficient reserves of energy to deal with emergency situations.

'Fitness' can therefore be defined as the ability to carry out effectively and efficiently some particular physical task or activity. 'Getting fitter' means advancing to a higher standard of fitness and being 'very fit' means possessing a standard of fitness better than most people. A sound standard of fitness normally corresponds with psychological well-being and freedom from disease. You do not have to be trained to the level of a champion athlete to appreciate the benefits of fitness. Once you have achieved a sound standard of fitness it does not take much to retain that standard, only three or four half-hour exercise sessions a week.

A sound standard of fitness is conducive to a zestful, productive life and enhances the possibility of reaching your full potential. Whatever your age, it is a highly desirable state to attain. If kept up through life, such an ongoing standard of fitness will also assist in the maintenance of bone health and the avoidance of bone-related disorders that can occur as you get older. Joint flexibility; reasonable muscle development; efficient lungs, heart and circulatory systems with reserve capability – these are important elements which contribute directly to the development of strength, stamina, speed, skill and suppleness, the components of fitness. In a while we will examine these components in more detail, but first of all, how fit are you?

HOW FIT ARE YOU?

Many people delude themselves as to how fit they are and how much exercise they take. As part of a recent Gallup survey[1] on personal fitness, the following question was put to interviewees: 'Would you describe yourself as a generally physically active person or not?' In response to the question nearly three out of four (72 per cent) admitted they were not. However, in response to the interviewer's question, 'If you have to choose between taking the lift or climbing three flights of stairs, which would you normally choose?' a completely different pattern of answers emerged. Only just over half (54 per cent) claimed they would normally take the stairs, with 46 per cent confession to normally taking the lift. Though two-thirds claimed to take regular exercise, when they were asked

---

[1] *Daily Telegraph*, 2 January 1996.

what form the exercise took, a large number and from all ages indicated that they regarded short walks – including walking the dog – as their primary exercise. The final question drew some degree of guilt from those sloth-inclined, for the question asked, 'Do you think you should take more exercise?' The answers showed that 60 per cent, made up of substantial majorities of all age groups, reckoned they should exercise more.

## A Simple Fitness Test

Health clubs and fitness centres offer elaborate fitness tests that combine an analysis of stamina, strength and suppleness and may produce an overall fitness rating. However, elaborate tests are not necessary if you just want to get some idea of your standard of basic fitness. The questionnaire below, reproduced with the permission of the Health Education and Sports Council, will help to give some guidance as to your degree of basic fitness.

Figure 1: Simple Fitness Test

| QUESTION | ANSWER YES | ANSWER NO |
| --- | --- | --- |
| 1. Do you quickly get out of breath walking uphill or even on the flat? | You need to improve our stamina. Walking more is the best way to start. | Good. If you want to build up even more stamina, try swimming or cycling. |
| 2. Do your legs ache or feel weak after you have climbed a couple of flights of stairs? | You need more leg strength. You could try the leg exercises on pages 221 and 222. | Good. Your legs are fairly strong. If you want them to get even stronger you could cycle or jog. |
| 3. Do you find it difficult to bend down and tie your shoelaces or put your socks or tights on? | You need to improve your suppleness. This book gives ideas for exercises and activities that help. | You are reasonably supple. It is worth making the effort to keep it that way as you get older. |
| 4. Do you find it difficult to comb the back of your hair or pull a jumper off? | You need more flexibility in your shoulder joints. | Good. Keep moving. |
| 5. Is it difficult to get out of an armchair or the bath? | You need to improve your suppleness and the strength in your arms and legs. | Good. You will find it a great advantage to work on your strength and suppleness, especially as you get older. |

There are three major qualities that contribute to general fitness: stamina, strength and suppleness. Each of these is examined below.

## Stamina

Stamina is the capacity to continue an activity for some period of time or to repeat a movement continuously. In simple terms it is the ability to 'keep going'. The length of time that we require to keep going determines the type of stamina required. It ranges from 'local muscular stamina' required to perform a series of powerful movements, such as press-ups (page 224) or wood chopping; to 'total stamina' where sustained effort is required over a prolonged period measured perhaps in hours, as with the long-distance runner, or even days or weeks, as in the case of the Arctic explorer.

Stamina depends on the efficiency of the lungs, heart, blood vessels and the working muscles. It is often referred to as 'aerobic', where the exercise will be moderately energetic, making you slightly out of breath, and will last for 20 minutes or more, during which you breathe in sufficient oxygen to provide an adequate supply to the working muscles, so withstanding the onset of fatigue.

Stamina applies to everyday life. It enables you to run or walk briskly some distance, as when in a hurry to catch a train, without getting tired or puffed. Training for stamina requires the lungs to work hard and the heart to pump efficiently over a sustained period. Stamina training is important, for it helps protect the heart against heart disease. The ability to perform exercise with minimum effort makes stamina the most important of the components of fitness.

Chapter 5 refers to exercising for stamina.

You need a certain degree of strength to carry out everyday activities that at times can be quite demanding and involve pushing, pulling and lifting – such as pushing a heavy shopping trolley uphill, pulling a garden roller or lifting heavy luggage at the airport. If you are in good shape it makes life easier and a person that has sufficient body strength has less chance of suffering from sprains and strains. Strength can be built up by increasing loads (see page 109).

Strength can be defined as the muscular force that we can apply with a single maximum effort against a resistance. It can be demonstrated in a number of ways:

STATIC STRENGTH involves 'isometric' resistance against a stationary load, for example holding up a heavy table in order to move a rug, or pushing against an equal force as in a rugby scrum. In isometric exercise muscles contract, without appreciable shortening, to exert tension or force against an immovable resistance.

DYNAMIC STRENGTH uses powerful 'isotonic' contractions to lift or move a load such as when lifting a heavy trunk or lifting and moving a piano. In isotonic exercise muscles shorten and lengthen to produce movement of body parts and is well demonstrated in weight training.

EXPLOSIVE STRENGTH involves powerful, fast muscular reactions as registered by the sprinter as he clears his blocks or by a high jumper. You would also need this type of strength in order to jump quickly out of the way of a car or cycle.

Chapter 6 refers to exercising for strength.

## Suppleness

Suppleness is demonstrated in the wide range of movement possible in a joint or at joint complexes. Suppleness affects bodily movement and posture. It contributes to fitness by determining the range limits through which limbs can or cannot move. Its presence or absence will very much influence a person's potential ability in a sport skill such as hurdling or gymnastics. In everyday life its presence helps you to avoid injuries when confronted by sudden bodily twists or distortion, such as when doing awkward jobs around the house or garden, or getting into and out from a small car.

Though it is possible to have stamina and strength but possess a body that is stiff and inflexible, the attainment and maintenance of suppleness, particularly with advancing years, is an important aspect of fitness and body efficiency. It should be noted that some forms of exercise can lead to muscles shortening, so, after exercising, it is important always to 'warm down' with a series of gentle stretching exercises.

Chapter 7 refers to exercising for suppleness.


### ADDITIONAL COMPONENTS OF FITNESS

The following qualities – speed and skill – are additional components of fitness to the three major components. Altogether they make for total fitness.


## Speed

Speed is the ability to move the body quickly. It is not restricted to the act of running fast but is displayed in the wider context of fast body movements, such as in the quick actions required of the squash and table-tennis player. Speed helps in our daily lives by providing the ability to run up and down stairs, or to chase and catch a child to avoid potential danger. It is possible to increase your running speed by a combination of training to improve technique, style and reaction time, together with strength training, aimed to give a greater power.

Chapter 8 refers to exercising for speed.

## Skill

Skill is the degree of proficiency that can be measured in a physical activity. It is an important aspect of every sport. We talk of tennis being a 'skilful' game. In this context skill is being used to describe an ongoing physical task made up of many individual techniques and movements. It is also possible to use the word to define a single movement, for example, trapping the ball in soccer.

Some skills can be broken down into a series of specific parts, each of which can be analysed: for instance, high jumping involves the run-up, take-off, movement over the bar, then the landing. Similarly, in the field of outdoor activities, the white-water kayak paddler aiming to 'break out' from an eddy behind rocks into a rapid will first pick up speed by paddling hard facing upstream; then, as the torrent hits his kayak, he will lean downstream, simultaneously supporting himself with his paddle on that side; and as the kayak turns he will paddle hard downstream to keep control of the kayak over the speed of the water. Such are the parts of this specific skill.

The requirement for a variety of basic skills is, for social, recreational or purely lifestyle reasons, with us throughout our lives – perhaps exemplified in the need to dance, swim, ride a bicycle, drive a car or shoot for sport (or to control game). Skill is a highly trainable aspect of fitness.

Chapter 9 refers to training for skill.

Though we have noted the merits of the three major components of fitness, i.e. strength, stamina and suppleness, plus the additional components of speed and skill, the importance is that they are often interrelated. Some activities, sports and vocations require more than one component. The beach lifeguard requires skill, stamina and strength to effect his rescue. The five events of the modern pentathlon – shooting, fencing, swimming, running and riding – embrace all five components of fitness. The hill farmer requires stamina and strength, as does the manual road worker. Perhaps to a lesser degree, the possession of stamina and strength are, of all the components, the most important for the average person.

# TWO

## Types and Effects of Exercise

- The Training Effect
    - Isotonic Exercise
    - Isometric Exercise
    - Anaerobic Exercise
    - Aerobic Exercise
    - Stretch Exercise
- The Interrelation of Exercise
- The Training Effect – Methods of Achieving
    - Pulse
    - Talking Test
- Effects of Exercise
    - Calories Burnt
    - Exercises and Appetite
- The Overload Principle
    - Progressive Overload Training
        - Degree of Resistance
        - Work Rate
        - Work Duration
        - Rest Intervals
    - Types of Overload
        - Stamina
        - Strength
        - Suppleness
        - Speed
        - Skill
- Muscle Structure

Exercise can take various forms and have different effects. The attainment of improved stamina, strength, speed, skill and suppleness requires, where possible, a defined intensity level and duration in order to initiate changes in body physiology. This is known as the 'training effect' and is essential in the development of overall, or endurance, fitness (see pages 29 and 53). Where strength is sought with the use of weights, the resistance involved and numbers of repetitions will determine whether strength is just improved, muscular endurance developed or maximum strength attained (see page 120).

There are five types of exercise, explained below together with methods of achieving the training effect.

Isotonic Exercise

Isotonic means 'equal tension'. It is a term used to describe a muscular contraction in which the muscle shortens or lengthens against a resistance or load, resulting in movement. The tension in an isotonic contraction is kept fairly constant while the muscle length changes. Traditional methods of strength training use isotonic exercise through the employment of suitably sized free weights, carrying out repeated movements. However, the use of training machines, where improved strength is achieved by working against hydraulic pistons, has become very popular. The effect is similar to that experienced with types of rowing machines where the more vigorous the effort made, the greater the hydraulic resistance experienced. Variable resistance machines are a form of machine that can vary the load placed upon the user.

Isometric Exercise

Isometric means 'equal measure'. It is a term used to describe a muscle contraction where the muscle length does not change, for the muscle contracts against an immovable resistance. This is demonstrated in the static strength required to hold a weight in a fixed position. Other examples are pushing out against a door frame, or clenching the fingers together in front of you at chest height with elbows up and pulling hard against your grip. Both exercises aim to strengthen the arms. There is therefore no limb movement in these exercises and the muscle length does not change due to the immovable resistance. Maximum force is developed in such an action but only in the one fixed position. Isometric exercises can increase the strength and size of individual skeletal muscles. Researchers claim that you must put maximum effort into exercise and hold the static tension for six seconds (pages 203ff. give essential progressions).

It is thought that isometric exercises have a beneficial effect for body-builders, but are also very valuable in the field of therapeutics and can be given to bedridden patients or immobile people so as to prevent muscles wasting away. The advantage of isometrics is that you need no equipment and it is possible to devise a simple series of exercises that will have an effect on body strength and muscle tone. They can make you feel good and can be performed in the office at lunchtime, or in the living-room. Try pulling your tummy in or tensing your thigh muscles when ironing or standing in the supermarket queue. However, isometrics have also proved of value to astronauts operating in their weightless state and have been used to maintain strength on long space voyages where other forms of exercise are not possible to perform.

It should be noted that isometrics have little training effect on the pulmonary and cardiovascular systems, for there is no significant increase in oxygen consumption. Isometric exercises tend to raise blood pressure during the actual exercise. Medical advice is best obtained before persons with blood pressure problems, or who are elderly, use these exercises.

Anaerobic Exercise

Anaerobic means 'without oxygen'. It is a form of exercise that can lead to the development of power, strength and muscular endurance. The primary objective is to increase the individual's capacity to tolerate 'oxygen debt'. This is the state arrived at when an intense activity demands exorbitant amounts of oxygen for short periods of time, so that the demands surpass the person's bodily capacity to supply sufficient oxygen, thus forcing him/her to stop and recover by elevating both breathing and heart rates. The length of the recovery period required is proportional to the size of the oxygen debt incurred and the degree of anaerobic fitness possessed by the person. According to Major Kenneth H. Cooper, MD, USAF, who produced one of the most important evaluations of physical fitness training ever with his 'aerobic system', anaerobic exercise fall into two types:

a. Firstly, exercise that demands a reasonable amount of oxygen, that will make you 'huff and puff', like running a comparatively short distance or swimming a few lengths. In these instances the exercise is cut short voluntarily and is over too quickly to have any real training benefits.

b. In the second type, the intensity of the exercise brings up oxygen demands that the body cannot meet, thus creating oxygen debt which must be paid back quickly. The exercise is cut short involuntarily due to the demands on the body. Examples of this type of exercise are sprinting 100 metres or 'all-out' sprint cycling. Such exercises are ideal for dedicated athletes to improve their speed and power, but are not necessary in an ordinary general fitness training programme, for they are over too quickly and therefore have little aerobic training effect.[1]

## Aerobic Exercise

Aerobic means 'with oxygen' and is the key to the development of cardio-respiratory endurance. Aerobic exercise is the type of exercise in which the oxygen demands on the body do not exceed the oxygen supply. This enables the exercise to be continued for long periods. Examples of aerobic

[1] K. H. Cooper, *Aerobics*.

exercise are cycling, walking, jogging and swimming carried out at a pace that stretches you a little, but permits sustained activity for some time (judged in many minutes or even hours).

Such intensity produces a training effect, so initiating physiological changes that will benefit the body, ensuring an increased consumption of oxygen and, as a result, improved endurance capability. The lungs will process more air with less effort, for the breathing rate will drop. The heart will become more efficient and stronger, increasing the stroke volume – that is, the amount of blood expelled from the heart with each beat, so pumping a greater amount of blood with fewer strokes and reducing the resting rate. The blood supply to muscles will also improve through an increase in the number and size of blood vessels, plus an increase in the total blood volume. Some authorities also believe that a healthy, efficient and well-conditioned heart can provide built-in protection against emotional crisis that could lead to the heart's deterioration and the possible onset of coronary heart disease.

## Stretch Exercise

Stretch exercises can be divided into active and passive exercise. With active stretch exercise the muscles contract isotonically to produce a full range of movement at specific joints, so as to exercise moderate force against the resistance of opposing muscles that are to be stretched or lengthened. This form of exercise is common in callisthenics (see pages 218–9, side bending). With passive stretch exercise the muscles contract isotonically to achieve a static held position, aiming to lengthen muscle groups (see page 146, shoulder stretch).

### THE INTERRELATION OF EXERCISE

Of the five concepts of exercise listed the most beneficial in terms of general fitness is that of aerobic exercise, which can ensure a training effect.

The training effect can be obtained through participating in what is known as the 'core' activities of running, walking, swimming or cycling. However, popular sports can also produce varying training effects and some of these will involve several concepts of exercise. If analysed, the game of hockey serves as a good example.

When taking a free hit or corner the hockey player firstly grips the stick tightly, tensing the arm muscles (isometric exercise). Now comes the drive – the short back-lift of the stick with the weight on the rear leg, the stroke then being made and controlled mainly by the forearms, the weight transferred to the forward leg as the ball is hit, the forward shoulder being kept up with the follow-through (isotonic exercise). The next stage involves anaerobic exercise as play commences and continues, for at times the player has to sprint, recover, then sprint again. The aerobic benefits will commence after play has been sustained for some time.

Conditioning exercises, or 'callisthenics', also defined as 'free-standing exercises' and developed into exercise done to music (the popular 'aerobic' dance-type movements) are set exercises that aim to improve strength, flexibility and posture. If they are carried out at a cadence that is not too energetic, so allowing exercising to continue for more than 20 minutes, they can produce a beneficial training effect. Progressive callisthenics are set exercises where the degree of difficulty is gradually increased to match the improvement of the individual.

THE TRAINING EFFECT – METHODS OF ACHIEVING

We have established that endurance is the most important element of general fitness. It concerns the efficiency with which the heart, lungs and circulatory system can provide oxygen and fuel to the body and eliminate waste products that would otherwise clog the muscles. Sustained activity, carried out for many minutes or even hours, can produce the training effect and will initiate changes to benefit the body. To recap, the lungs will become capable of processing more air with less effort, giving increased oxygen consumption. The heart will become stronger and more efficient, being able to pump more blood with fewer strokes. The blood supply to the muscles will improve and the total blood volume will increase. Dependent on your condition, it can take time to achieve a training effect: first of all you have to get the body systems to work so that the lungs are puffing and the heart pumping, but progressions must be graded to avoid over-taxing the body.

## Pulse

Though it is not necessary to take your pulse rate when exercising, some people like to do so, for your pulse is a good indicator of overall fitness. The pulse rate is also a useful guide to the level of activity that will have an aerobic training effect. The resting pulse rate registers your heart rate when you are not physically active and is usually best recorded before getting out of bed. As you become fitter and the heart becomes a more efficient pump, the effect of exercise is to reduce the resting pulse rate. Fitness training can also reduce the pulse recovery time, that is, the time it takes for the pulse to return to normal after a set exercise session.

To find your pulse, place the tips of the middle three fingers of your right hand gently over the radial pulse on the thumb side of your left wrist with the palm facing up (figure 2). Reverse the procedure if you are left handed. The pulse can also be taken at the neck over the carotid artery located below your ear lobe near the angle of the jaw. Count the beat for ten seconds, remembering to start at 'nought' and not at 'one' for otherwise you will make your pulse too fast. Now multiply by six to determine the beats per minute. Checking on your pulse rate immediately after a bout of set energetic exercises, and again after resting for two or three minutes, will give some idea of how your heart is reacting to endurance training and serve as a useful guide to progress.

It is generally believed that a safe maximum heart rate (MHR) for a person in sound health is deduced by subtracting your age from 210. For example, in the case of a 40-year-old person this would give 170 beats per minute as the safe maximum. To obtain a good training effect the heart should be working at around three quarters of the theoretical maximum.

This is known as the 'training heart rate' (THR). In the case of the 40-year-old it will give a THR of about 127 beats per minute. When beginning an aerobic programme it is advisable to work initially at the lower end of the range, at a THR that is about 60 per cent of the MHR.

Figure 2: Locating the Pulse

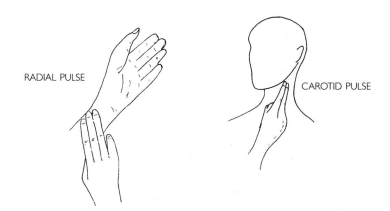

The duration of the activity is relevant and the heart rate should be maintained at its training rate for at least 20 minutes. Should the exercise not be vigorous enough to attain the THR, but is still demanding oxygen, the exercise will still produce aerobic benefits if sustained for an extended period. An example would be a long steady walk where the heart rate would not usually exceed 85 to 100 beats per minute. The taking of pulse readings can serve to encourage interest and further effort.

For those who are keen to keep a constant check on their heart rate so as to attain an optimum training effect, a heart-rate monitor comprising a wrist-watch-type display unit and a chest transmitter held in place by a belt will provide the information you want. They are particularly useful for the outdoor exerciser. Polar and York are two of the well-known brand names in this field. Some of the modern training machines (see pages 228ff.) incorporate pulse sensors that can be attached to the ear lobe or fingertip, or placed over the heart, and record the pulse rate on the visual computer screen of the machine.

Talking Test

Some researchers believe that people have the ability to estimate their levels of exertion and that this is more practical and less time consuming than pulse taking. Common sense, and the knowledge that you would be doing too much if you reached a state of breathlessness where you could not talk to a partner (real or imagined) or whistle, can ensure that any harmful strain is avoided. If you cannot talk or whistle then the effort being made is more likely anaerobic and of greater intensity than necessary for safe training. Beginners would be unwise to continue at this level. But one further word about the 'talking test': if you do get breathless, slow down until conversation is possible – you will get fitter by doing so.

Finally, and most important, before embarking on any programme that will subject the body to unaccustomed stress, take note of the medical precautions on page 61.

EFFECTS OF EXERCISE – CALORIES BURNT AND APPETITE

Calories Burnt

Whether people gain or lose weight depends on the balance between energy consumed in food and the energy used in living. This is measured in 'calories'. A calorie is defined as a unit of work or energy equating to the amount of heat required to raise the temperature of one gram of water one degree centigrade. When the body is in calorie balance the energy intake and output are equal and the body weight remains constant. Eat more calories than you use and weight will be gained; use more than you eat and weight will be lost. Being active is not only good for the heart and circulation, it can use up many calories, which results in weight being controlled.

People vary in the amount of energy they use when doing similar activities. The figures opposite give a general outline as to the amount of energy used daily and may help you calculate a personal daily diet/exercise programme.

If you need to lose weight it is best to obtain expert advice

Figure 3: Daily Activities – Calories Used

| ACTIVITY | CALORIES USED PER MINUTE |
|---|---|
| Sleeping | 1 |
| Sitting, standing and sedentary office work | 1.5 |
| Vigorous housework | 4 |
| Slow walking | 4 |
| Golf | 4 |
| Easy cycling | 5 |
| Brisk walking | 5 |
| Fast walking | 6 |
| Field games | 6.5 |
| Swimming | 7 |
| Tennis | 7 |
| Brisk cycling | 7.5 |
| Strenuous work | 10 |
| Squash | 11 |
| Jogging | 12 |
| Running | 20 |

from a dietician and, if need be, the guidance of your doctor. The easiest way can be to reduce your intake of high-fat foods, as each gram of fat supplies nine calories, which is twice the amount supplied by one gram of protein or sugar or starch. Low-fat foods that can assist weight reduction are fruit, vegetables (cooked without fat), rice, pasta, wholemeal bread, oat products, poultry, fish, lean meat and low-fat milk.

Exercise and Appetite

When we take exercise it causes an increase in our metabolic rate, that is the complex chemical changes where by the body converts food into energy. Exercise can take away the appetite, for it is suppressed by the appetite depressant effects of a chemical substance produced in the body for 60–90 minutes after vigorous physical exercise. This is accompanied by a rise in body temperature, plus other chemical changes. A reduced food requirement and intake, combined with a higher metabolic rate brought about by exercise, can result in the body weight dropping to a lower level. Further exercise undertaken combined with a calorie-controlled intake can result in the breakdown of fat stores, thus maintaining the lower body weight.

Exercise has an ongoing reaction. For the next two hours after a two-hour brisk walk you will continue to burn double the amount of the calorie normally burnt by the body. More demanding exercise, such as running for half an hour, can result in the increase in calorie consumption continuing for five to six hours after the exercise has finished. Sustained exercise, even of a modest intensity, if maintained over a period will burn calories. If the intensity of the exercise is increased, so will the number of calories burnt. The following gives a broad example of the approximate number of calories burnt while walking for 30 minutes at 2 mph (slow pace) then for two hours, in comparison with those burnt when walking at an increased speed of 4 mph (fast pace) over the same time spans.

| SPEED | CALORIES BURNT (APPROXIMATE) | |
| --- | --- | --- |
| | *30 mins* | *2 hours* |
| Slow pace (2 mph) | 120–145 | 480–580 |
| Fast pace (4 mph) | 180–215 | 720–860 |

The safest way of losing weight is to do so gradually, aiming perhaps to lose no more than two pounds a week. A combination of dieting and exercise could achieve this, as a reduction of 500 calories per day could shed a pound of fat in a week (approximately 3,500 calories), plus 500 calories burnt per day through exercise.

THE OVERLOAD PRINCIPLE

One of the phenomena of the human body is its ability to adjust to the demands of physical stress placed upon it. A person's level of fitness is imaged in the specific adaptations made to their shape, weight, body flexibility and movement, related to the level of physical activity habitually encountered in their work or leisure pursuits. The body can also respond by adapting to meet the demands of planned diverse physical activity. It may register an improvement in muscle strength, endurance, speed, flexibility and co-ordination, dependent on the type of activity being undertaken and the intensity and progressions entailed. Conversely, inactivity will produce adverse changes in these areas and a decline in the body's efficiency.

Perhaps one of the earliest examples of the effects of increased exercise benefiting the body was demonstrated by Milo of Crotona, the Greek wrestler of ancient times. It is said that Milo trained by carrying a calf around on his shoulders in order to increase his strength. As the calf grew into a small bull and Milo's burden dramatically increased, it resulted in his body adapting and becoming fitter and stronger. This concept of progressively increasing the load and its training effect is known as the 'overload principle'. It can be defined as 'the application of any demand or resistance that is greater than those levels normally encountered in daily life'. The degree of intensity with which the system is overloaded will affect the rate at which physiological adaptations take place. The closer the overload is to maximum, the greater the physiological improvement, provided that the overload is applied in gradual progressions and can be tolerated by the body – for it takes time for the human body to adapt to additional exercise without experiencing fatigue or excessive muscle soreness. Below a certain stress level a person will show no improvement and merely maintain his current level of physical fitness.

## Progressive Overload Training

The aim of a fitness programme can be an improvement in one or more of the components of fitness, i.e. stamina, strength, suppleness, speed or skill. The result will be seen in physiological changes to the body achieved by progressive increases in the intensity of the overload, applied in the following ways:

DEGREE OF RESISTANCE The amount of resistance is increased by lifting heavier weights or loads by applying greater force. An example would be to add a few more weights on the bar when doing bench presses or, when doing step-ups, carry a dumb-bell in each hand and then gradually increase the weight.

WORK RATE The work rate is increased by performing the exercise or task in a shorter period of time. Instead of walking a mile in 20 minutes, cover the distance in 15 minutes.

WORK DURATION The work period is increased but the same work intensity is retained. An example would be to increase your 4 mph walk to cover five miles at the same speed in one hour and 15 minutes.

REST INTERVALS The rest periods taken between training repetitions or set exercise periods is reduced, for instance when carrying out 'scout pace' (see page 76) – perhaps comprising walking for 800 yards, then jogging for 200 yards, gradually reducing the walking phase to 400 yards and increasing the jogging phase to 300 yards. When doing step-ups in three sets perhaps of 20 reps, reduce the rest period between each set (see page 116).

## Types of Overload

Training for any of the components of fitness tends to be highly specific, but the principles of overload can be applied to each of the components. When planning a training programme it is necessary to define clearly the areas that you need to improve and the type of overload required. The following types of overload are used to bring about improvements in:

STAMINA through increased duration, so increasing total repetitions but maintaining the same work rate, or by decreasing rest time between set work periods.

STRENGTH through increased resistance by increased weights lifted, or increased muscle tension exerted.

SUPPLENESS through resistance by force exerted by opposing muscle groups to produce movement, or by static body positions held, aiming to stretch or lengthen muscles.

SPEED through increasing the rate of work; also by decreasing the rest time between work periods. To this training is added a degree of strength training.

SKILL through duration, initially by short practice sessions with suitable rest periods. These are more beneficial in learning a skill than long practice sessions with short rest periods. Once the time intervals of the different portions of the movement are perceived and undertaken and the skill correctly performed, you can gradually reduce the resting periods and increase the speed of the skill and its repetitions, but must always carefully monitor technique.

## MUSCLE STRUCTURE

All our movements are achieved through muscular action. Muscles are bundles of fibres through which run blood vessels and nerves. Muscle fibres in turn are composed of smaller fibrils, each packed with muscle protein which is arranged to overlap other fibrils. They initiate the force in muscle contractions by means of a ratchet-like action. The size of the muscles is popularly believed to determine a person's strength. This, in some cases, can be misleading since muscle bulk can be made up of non-contractile tissue, that is, connective tissue that does not provide power. Such examples can be seen in the muscle bulk of some body-builders and brought about by 'pumping' methods that result in increased blood vessels and blood in their muscles.

The size of actual muscle tissue is dependent on firstly the number of fibres within the muscle and secondly the thickness of the individual fibres. There are a number of different types of fibres within a muscle. Some are known as 'fast twitch' fibres which are thick, white and have a highly developed anaerobic system. When the nervous system signals the muscle to contract, the fast twitch fibres respond very quickly and simultaneously, being capable of generating great force.

Other fibres are thinner and have a well-developed aerobic energy processing system. These are 'slow twitch' fibres. They are red and, when stimulated, respond more slowly. The fast twitch fibres are essential for explosive movements, such as sprint starts, throwing events and weight-lifting. They do not rely on the continuous delivery of oxygen to the tissue and therefore work anaerobically. The slow twitch fibres are essential for endurance, such as long-distance running and cycling. Slow twitch fibres work aerobically, requiring a steady supply of oxygen to convert sugar and fat into energy.

The proportion of fast twitch and slow twitch fibres in muscles varies from person to person and is determined by heredity. This helps explain why some people have the innate ability to sprint well while others are successful at endurance events.

# THREE

## Exercise and Bone Health

- Types of Bone
  - Compact or Cortical Bone
  - Spongy or Trabecular Bone
- Osteoporosis
- The Importance of Exercise to Bone Health
  - Childhood and Adolescence
  - Types of Activity
  - Exercise Programmes
- Before You Start

Bone strength is essential to the performance of everyday living and to the carrying out of all the demanding tasks that the human body must, at times, fulfil.

The skeleton gives shape to the body, supports its weight, protects vital organs, permits movement and gives points of attachment for muscles to act as levers. Bones also act as a storehouse, for 99 per cent of the body's calcium is contained in bone.

### TYPES OF BONE

There are two types of bone within the body:

COMPACT OR CORTICAL BONE is a close-weave material which looks solid and dense. It is to be found especially in the limbs and predominates in the shafts of the long bones. Cortical bone constitutes 80 per cent of the total skeletal mass.

SPONGY OR TRABECULAR BONE comprises a lace-type, more porous composition and is present especially in the vertebrae of the spine, but is also found in the pelvis and other flat bones and in the ends of long bones. Though having a delicate appearance, trabecular bone is very strong.

Both cortical and trabecular bone is made up of three different components. These are:

a. The framework of the bone, known as the matrix.
b. The mineral element, where calcium is stored, that makes the bone rigid, hard and strong.
c. Osteoblast (bone-forming) cells and osteoclast (bone-resorbing) cells, that in normal healthy bone work together in a fine balance, allowing adequate new bone to replace that gobbled up by the bone-resorbing cells. It is believed that with the disease of osteoporosis the balance becomes disturbed: the action of the bone-forming cells slows down, or that of the bone-resorbing cells speeds up, or both occur at once.

OSTEOPOROSIS

Osteoporosis is the most common disorder of the skeleton. At one time osteoporosis was considered purely a women's disease, but males can often display similar characteristics. Affecting one in four women and one in twelve men, it results in a reduction in both the amount and strength of bone tissue, so that the affected part or parts of the skeleton are abnormally susceptible to fractures. The most obvious manifestation of osteoporosis is a fracture, usually in the vertebrae, wrist or hip (figure 4).

Bone mass begins to decline around the age of 30 in women and 50 in men.[1] Trabecular bone is lost faster than cortical bone, due to its large lattice-type surface area which renders it more vulnerable when bone loss takes place. This, it is believed, results in the onset of osteoporosis in the spine earlier than in

[1] Office of Health Economics, *Osteoporosis*.

40

the hip. The avoidance of brittle bones is highly desirable. It has been found that certain types of exercise can play an important role in helping to maintain bone strength and bone health; also in avoiding the degeneration of bone through the loss of bone density, a cause of vulnerability to bone fractures.

Ageing is one of the most important factors in bone loss. By the age of 70 bone mass may have declined by as much as 30 per cent or more in women, less in men.[1] Therefore low bone mass is almost universal among the elderly, though it should be noted that there are also some elderly who do not show any marked difference in bone mass, nor do they fracture their bones. In women, osteoporosis can affect three age groups. Firstly, women around 35 years who have a family history of osteoporosis. Secondly, it is common after the menopause and is seen after the age of 50. The third age group occurs at the older age of 70 and 75; men can also be affected at this age.

While the tendency for this disability can be inherited, it can also be affected by sex and race. White women are more at risk than white men. Black men and women have a lower incidence of osteoporosis. As black people have a greater bone mass and greater bone density they experience fewer vertebrae fractures than white people. Black people also tend to have larger muscles than whites and consequently the greater stress imposed on their bones by normal activity results in larger

Figure 4: Osteoporosis

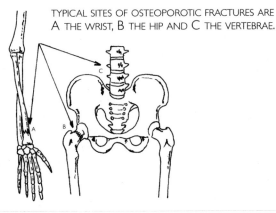

TYPICAL SITES OF OSTEOPOROTIC FRACTURES ARE A THE WRIST, B THE HIP AND C THE VERTEBRAE.

[1] Office of Health Economics, op. cit.

bones. Other factors that may increase the possibility of osteoporosis include smoking, diets low in calories and calcium, an excessive alcohol intake and certain medications such as corticosteroids. A sedentary lifestyle can also accelerate the ageing process and with it bone loss.

After the age of about 35 women's bones may become thinner due to the loss of calcium. The loss accelerates after the menopause, when oestrogen levels fall due to the reduction in oestrogen secretion from the ovaries, and can result in osteoporosis and the risk of fractures. This body imbalance can also be experienced by women ballet dancers and women endurance athletes who, due to their abnormally low oestrogen levels, stop menstruating – with the result of reduced bone density at a degree similarly encountered in post-menopausal women.[1] This is thought to be due to intensive training and calorie restriction, which causes changes in body composition and a reduction in body fat. Psychological stress can also contribute, particularly in the case of competitive athletes.

It is possible that an extra intake of the mineral calcium, which is essential to building strong bones in childhood, will help offset the loss of bone density encountered in most menopausal women when oestrogen levels drop. Medical research has concluded that hormone replacement therapy (HRT) treatment within the first years after the menopause can delay or prevent osteoporosis and HRT is known to stop bone loss and prevent fractures. Exposure to the sun in moderation has its benefits, for it allows the body to make vitamin D which is needed by the body to absorb calcium.[2]

It is estimated that osteoporosis causes approximately 1.5 million fractures each year, with fractures of the hip and wrist being particularly common in older women – resulting, for many, in lack of mobility. Other serious complications of osteoporosis are fractures of the spinal column vertebrae that can result in the shortening of a person's actual height. In other cases an exaggerated curvature can develop, causing what is known in the female as the 'dowager's hump'.

[1] R.L. Wolman, 'ABC of Sports Medicine', *British Medical Journal*, vol. 309, 6 August 1994.

[2] A. Fairney and J. Wilson, *Osteoporosis – Booklet for Patients*.

Bones need movement and the pull of tendons and muscles exercising against the force of gravity to maintain their strength. Exercise also increases the blood flow to the bones thus bringing in necessary bone-building nutrients. However, to guard against osteoporosis, any exercise planned needs to be weight bearing. Research shows that such exercise may stimulate bone-forming cells to make new bone. The skeletal response to stress is greatest at the site of maximum stress. For example, a tennis player's playing arm can be up to 30 per cent denser in bone structure than the non-playing arm. Runners have increased bone density in the calcaneous (heel), femoral shaft (thigh) and spine. Rowers display an increase in spinal bone density.[1]

## Childhood and Adolescence

It is believed that habitual physical activity maintains and increases the mineral content of the skeleton and this effect is apparent at every age.[2] The fact is of particular relevance to children as the skeletal bone mass increases during childhood and adolescence. The beneficial effects of exercise and suitable diet are of primary importance during this period of growth and beyond, for peak bone mass may not be reached until 30 years. The greater the bone mineral density at the end of the growing period, the later in life it may be that bones degenerate to a point where there could be the risk of fractures. Active children and active young adults have denser bones than those of comparable age who do little exercise. They are therefore off to a good start in life. It would be reasonable to predict that those who do little exercise at this time of life may be disadvantaged in years to come. The future health of the young is, I believe, under threat. The changing patterns of school and family life are not to their advantage. There is little opportunity for the young to take part in

[1] Wolman, op. cit.

[2] Fentem, op. cit.

dynamic PE games at school. Many do not involve themselves in the active enjoyable play once associated with children: they take little exercise but spend much time watching television, playing video games or using computers. Added to these factors can be a diet of unhealthy fast-food. They are the ingredients that could, in later life, lead to medical problems and the possibility of osteoporosis. Bone density does not plateau until after peak bone mass is achieved. In females, age-related bone loss begins between 35 and 40. Following the menopause women experience an accelerated bone loss for several years; but research into women of all ages from 20 to 80, who exercised three times a week or more, showed a higher bone density than women of a similar age who did not exercise.[1]

## Types of Activity

Activities that are of an aerobic nature, that is, exercise that can be sustained for a long period such as swimming, moderate-pace walking and cycling, may certainly improve cardio-respiratory (heart and lungs) fitness. However, as they do not involve substantial weight-bearing exercise, they have but a limited overall effect on the promotion of bone density in comparison with some other exercises. They are known as 'low-impact' activities. Such activities are of course excellent forms of core fitness training. They may also be suitable for people who have joint problems, or who are very much overweight and require non-jarring motion.

In order to have the most beneficial effect upon the skeletal system by promoting bone density and therefore bone strength, activities undertaken need to be vigorous and, as stated, involve weight-bearing exercises. Such 'high-impact' activities include vigorous walking, jogging, running, weight training, racket games, hopping, skipping, stair climbing and vigorous dancing. Examples of benefits of high-impact activities are:

---

[1] Fentem, op. cit.

| PHYSICAL ACTIVITY/GAME | LOCATION OF BONE DENSITY INCREASES |
|---|---|
| Running/jogging/skipping | Heel, shin, thigh bones and spine. |
| Squash/tennis | Bones of dominant arm, spine and legs. |
| Volleyball/netball/basketball | Heel, legs, spine (and arms to a lesser degree). |

Often the preferred programme of an active person may be based on a low-impact type of aerobic exercise, such as moderate-pace walking. It is therefore worth adding to this programme an element of bone-stressing, to assist bone health. This can be achieved by including some high-impact activity which could take the form of astride jumping, skipping, or running on the spot, carried out at the completion of your walk prior to warming-down.

As stated, exercise that entails repetitive stress loading on a part of the skeleton will tend to increase bone density in that part. As bone mass appears to increase significantly in areas exposed to the pull of tendons and muscles, physical activity directed to those areas vulnerable to fractures – such as the spine, hip and wrist – can help minimise or even prevent fractures.[1] This should be done under medical direction if weakness is already present. Furthermore, exercise that aims to stimulate bone formation should be diverse, vigorous and repetitive.[2]

The value of exercise in this field is documented. Carefully monitored patients were required to hop as high as possible for several seconds each day, morning and evening; others were called upon to squeeze a tennis ball tightly three times, twice a day. In both instances there was a considerable increase in the bone density in the bones under stresss.[3] Aerobic training that involves continuous repetitive movement, such as running or jogging for some distance, will lead after several months of training to appreciable increases in bone density, particularly in the spine. Walking, dancing and running all affect and benefit the hips as a weight-bearing part of the body. Strength training, where controlled stress loading is imposed upon part of the

---

[1] Office of Health Economics, op. cit.

[2] National Osteoporosis Society, *Exercise and Physiotherapy in the Prevention and Treatment of Osteoporosis.*

[3] A. Ripley and L. Ferris, *Forty Plus.*

body to build up muscular strength, will also increase bone density. Research in America published by the *Journal of Orthopedic Research* found that those women who remained physically fit after the menopause, or after the age of 50, had greater bone strength and density than women of a similar age who took no exercise. When compared with inactive women aged 50 to 75, fit women of the same age had greater spine and arm bone density; and they registered bone density readings that were the same as women 10 to 15 years younger.

Exercise may reduce the risk of osteoporosis even with people in their 80s. In addition it improves alertness, also muscle tone and balance, so lessening the chances of falls and fractures.[1] When age and fitness permit, the disease of osteoporosis can be slowed and even halted by regular high-impact exercise combined with a high calcium diet. Such a pattern of exercise and diet also ensures that if a fit woman had the misfortune to break bones, her bones will unite and heal quicker than those of an unfit woman. Exercise can also improve posture by keeping the back and tummy muscles tight and the shoulders held back. It's also good for your self-image.

Chapter 10 gives a variety of exercises that can be pursued at home. Many of the exercises contribute to the promotion of bone health and as a guide I have outlined their approximate values in the promotion of bone health as 'high', 'medium' or 'low'.

## Exercise Programmes

The amount of exercise we take as children and in adolescence can therefore determine the degree of bone health we will enjoy in later life and can relate to our quality of life in middle and old age. The amount of exercise taken by women in their 30s whose families have a history of osteoporosis can also be very important. R.L. Wolman, writing in the *British Medical Journal*, records that intensive aerobic training can paradoxically lead to a fall in bone density caused by low oestrogen levels.[2] The exercise and oestrogen levels of a woman

[1] Wolman, op. cit.

[2] Ibid.

in her 20s and 30s may be very important in determining her eventual risk of developing osteoporosis. As regards older women it is stated by the Office of Health Economics (OHE), as researched by B. Krolner, that 30 minutes' moderate exercise per day such as walking, jogging or dancing, will reduce bone loss in post-menopausal women.[1] One hour's walking twice a week for eight months was found to increase the bone mineral content of the spine by 3.5 per cent.

The OHE stresses the danger of exercise being incorrectly performed, thus increasing the risk of accident and fractures. Exercises that are over-intensive and impose too much strain obviously have their dangers, but the OHE concludes that, apart from the time spent on exercise there are few costs involved and the benefits of gentle, careful exercise outweigh any associated risks.

## BEFORE YOU START

Medical precautions relating to exercise are noted on page 61. If you have a non-active lifestyle, have already experienced fractures or pain, or have a medical condition which may make some types of exercise unsuitable, consult your GP or hospital doctor before you start exercising. In such circumstances, before embarking on any training programme that you are not used to, seek confirmation that the activities you select are suitable for your medical circumstances and age. Begin exercising very gently and gradually build up the level of exertion. Generally speaking, any increase in the intensity of the exercise should be by small stages. These slow, gentle progressions are particularly important for the elderly or unfit. The British Medical Journal records that most people over the age of 50, however sedentary their life pattern has been, can benefit from physical activity provided progress is slow and cautious.[2]

Participation in such activities or exercises will give additional benefits including a feeling of well-being, a higher standard of fitness and an improved lifestyle. Hopefully it could form a new pattern of life.

[1] Office of Health Economics, op. cit.

[2] Fentem, op. cit.

# FOUR

# Getting Started

- Exercise and Body Types
    Endomorph
    Mesomorph
    Ectomorph
- Aims and Objectives
- Initial Fitness – Core Activities
- Practical Points
    Training Time – How Long?
      How Often?
    An Exercise Programme
    When to Exercise
    Warming Up and Warming Down
    Rest and Recovery
    Over-exercising and When to Stop
    Symptoms of Over-exercising
    A Fitness Diary/Log
- Medical Precautions
- Exercise Tips

It has long been recognised that there is a definite relationship between body build and physical aptitude. The type of body that a person inherits makes him/her more suitable for some activities than for others. Recognition of relative fitness and aptitude ensures that individuals may select activities they can enjoy to the full and also achieve success.

Many attempts have been made to classify body types. Way back in 400 BC Hippocrates distinguished two extremes of body type: *Habitus Phthysicus* (long, thin) and *Habitus Appoplecticus* (short, thick). Halle in 1797 defined four types: abdominal, muscular, thoracic (long chest, slender), and nervous. However, the most significant contribution in this area was made by W.H. Sheldon and his co-workers who, in the 1940s, concluded that there were three distinct body classifications: 'endomorph' (round, soft, fat), 'mesomorph' (husky, muscular, athletic), and 'ectomorph' (thin, frail, slender).

To cover the wide variations within these extremes Sheldon appraised each of the three components on a seven-point scale. The body type of a person is designated by three component numbers. The endomorphic component is always given first, then the mesomorphic, then the ectomorphic. These points were arrived at from photographs taken of each subject from the front, side and back, plus a height/weight index and body measurements. An extreme endomorph would be rated 711, the extreme mesomorph as 171 and the extreme ectomorph as 117. But extremes are rare and such ratings as 533 and 443 would be typical. The dominant physical features, health characteristics and exercise potential of the three body types are as follows:

Figure 5: The Extremes of Human Physique

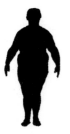 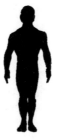 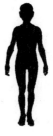

ENDOMORPH      MESOMORPH      ECTOMORPH

## Endomorph

DOMINANT PHYSICAL FEATURES Ponderous, soft, fatty physique. Short, thick neck. Large head, abdomen and chest. Well-rounded shoulders.

HEALTH CHARACTERISTICS Prone to excess fat and consequently organic disorders. Men of such physique are not suited for hard physical work and are apt to avoid such tasks, so aggravating the tendency to obesity.

EXERCISE POTENTIAL Likely to achieve physical and mental satisfaction from activities such as swimming, cycling, sailing, bowling, fishing, camping, archery and shooting.

## Mesomorph

DOMINANT PHYSICAL FEATURES Strong, well-developed musculature. Strong bones. Broad shoulders. Deep chest and narrow waist. Little superfluous fat.

HEALTH CHARACTERISTICS Usually energetic people and capable of a greater physical work output than either of the other two groups. Provided they do not over-train, they suffer few ailments. In middle age they need to take care not to overeat and under-exercise which can result in a tendency to put on weight and so adopt some endomorphic characteristics.

EXERCISE POTENTIAL Excel in sports that require strength, speed and power, such as sprinting, throwing and major body contact team games which involve tackling and charging, e.g. soccer and rugby.

## Ectomorph

DOMINANT PHYSICAL FEATURES Angular, fragile profile. Thin, long limbs, trunk and neck. Limited musculature. Ribs prominent and little body fat. Small joints and supporting tissue.

HEALTH CHARACTERISTICS Usually long lived and enjoy a good standard of health provided they have a balanced diet, have adequate exercise and are not exposed to extremes of cold or dampness where they can suffer due to their lack of insulating body fat.

EXERCISE POTENTIAL Light physical structure normally renders them unsuitable for activities that require great strength, body contact or involvement in throwing events. However, they are likely to achieve physical and mental satisfaction from such games and sports as cricket, tennis, distance walking and running.

After the age of about nine years, fat in females accounts for a higher percentage of total body weight than in males. Women therefore have a tendency to be more endomorphic in their body structure and are, at all ages, heavier in proportion to stature. There is also a tendency for the body fat of both males and females to increase with age. Throughout life your basic body type remains relatively constant, but marked changes can be made within your body type. They can occur particularly in regard to the most unstable component, fat, normally with an increase in weight brought about by too great a calorie intake and too little exercise. Changes can also take place in muscle bulk through a reduction in muscle size due to inactivity, or an increase achieved by regular exercise.

Regardless of your basic body type, it is possible through awareness and action to achieve a desirable level of health and fitness, a better physical appearance, enjoyment and a feeling of well-being, from participation in the sort of exercise most suited to you.

## AIMS AND OBJECTIVES

It is important that any initial exercise experience is refreshing and relaxing. The term 'programme' can be misleading and off-putting. An exercise programme for some may consist of a daily cycle to collect the newspaper, walking the dog some distance twice a day, or a workout with improvised weights in the garage. For others it may comprise a detailed plan involving aerobic, strength and flexibility exercises, eventually culminating in participation in a competitive sport.

Ideally an exercise programme should be tailored to each person's requirements and take into account such factors as age, body type, health, physical fitness, lifestyle, fitness aims, degree of self-motivation and facilities available. Aims can vary. You may exercise to improve your image or lifestyle, to become competitive, perhaps to enjoy company, or to improve your skill; or just to feel good, be healthier and keep the waistline under control. Maybe there are some attractive members in the local tennis club – time to get fit and take up the game! For others, there are the delights of those country walks and feeling pure air entering your lungs, the tingle of the wind and rain on your face, the silence that dissolves all sense of time, and with it the stresses of daily life.

When planning to get fit you should have three objectives. Firstly, aim to get fit as soon as is practicable. Secondly, have an ongoing uninterrupted plan. Thirdly, achieve your desired standard of fitness by following a schedule that avoids injury. Your guiding principles should be 'train don't strain'.

You may be starting from a low standard of fitness. If so, your initial improvement may be comparatively rapid, but once you become fitter you may not be able to keep up the same rate of progress Don't be disappointed if this is the case for, as you exercise, your fitness will continue to improve steadily.

Younger people in their teens or 20s who are not suffering from weight problems can, with a carefully contrived programme, bring themselves from a state of inactivity to a fair standard of fitness within eight to twelve weeks. Those who are in their 40s may take twice as long and people in their 60s even longer, perhaps eight to ten months or more. However long it takes to get fit, bear in mind that exercise should always be enjoyed rather than endured. What is important is that you seek out a pattern of physical activity that fits your lifestyle, stretches you a little, but is enjoyable to undertake. Once you have done this, set yourself realistic targets and obtain the satisfaction of achieving them.

## INITIAL FITNESS – CORE ACTIVITIES

The best way to get fit initially is to concentrate on one or more of the core activities of walking, running, cycling and swimming. They are highly aerobic activities that develop endurance, are readily available to most people, can be easily practised and are time efficient. Once a fair standard of basic fitness has been achieved through participation in core activities, you can continue with these activities in order to retain or to develop your standard of fitness further. There are many other activities and sports that will keep you fit and the aerobic values of these are recorded in figure 8 on page 67.

PRACTICAL POINTS

As indicated in chapter 1, fitness is a specific quality that can relate to a particular activity, task or sport. If you are exercising for strength then you need to work the relevant muscles; if you are exercising for endurance then you must exercise the heart and lungs to have that aerobic effect. The body will adapt to the type of training imposed upon it but, as you become fitter, the original exercise training level will no longer be intense enough to bring about those physiological changes that will increase your standard of fitness. In general, the achievement of greater fitness should involve better rather than more training. In many cases exercise sessions should become progressively more intense. Performance ought to get quicker, or involve greater resistance, rather than just become longer.

To achieve our aims a number of factors need to be considered in any exercise programme. For how long and how often should we exercise? What format should an exercise programme take? Is there a best time of day to exercise? How important is the warm-up and warm-down? How important is rest after exercise? What are the symptoms of over-exercising? These practical points are discussed in the following paragraphs.

Training Time – How Long? How Often?

Generally speaking, once fit you should exercise at least three times a week, for approximately 20 to 30 minutes each session, spread out so as to exercise every other day. The actual exercise time in minutes is linked to the minimum amount of exercise that is required to produce significant improvements in aerobic fitness – sometimes referred to as the 'training threshold'. For the development of aerobic fitness the training threshold is regarded by some authorities as a minimum of 20 minutes of physical effort that would generate a heart rate of between 60 and 80 per cent of the MHR. In order to maintain the training effect, exercise must be carried out regularly.

There are other benefits to such frequent exercise carried out at a similar intensity. Regular training sessions involving jogging, running, swimming, cycling or dancing; games and sports carried out for 30 minutes; brisk walking for about an hour – all these, practised three or more times a week, can make significant changes to the composition of the body. Body fat will be reduced and muscle mass increased. In the earlier stages of exercising body weight may remain constant, though weight loss should occur as training continues, provided the calorie intake is controlled.

Beginners would be unwise to exercise for more than 30 minutes at an intensity that has a training effect. Initial sessions should be about 15 to 20 minutes and at a heart rate best kept at no more than 60 per cent of the MHR. If necessary, divide the sessions into parts, with recovery periods of a minute or two between more intense phases of activity.

Within reason, provided the individual is sufficiently fit and prepared, the longer the exercise session the greater the aerobic benefit, though beyond an hour the return is less. Experts also believe that a regular weekly aerobic exercise programme of three to five sessions lasting 20 to 30 minutes, practised at an intensity that has an aerobic training effect, will help to reduce the risk of coronary heart disease.

An Exercise Programme

A general exercise programme can comprise four parts. The first part warms the body up in preparation for the more strenuous exercise to come. The second part of the programme, the aerobic training phase, aims to improve the efficiency of the heart and lungs to be followed by a muscle conditioning phase. The programme would end with a warm-down and relaxation phase. An example of a general exercise programme based on this format is as follows:

Figure 6: Example of a General Exercise Programme

| PHASE | EXERCISE | APPROXIMATE TIME |
|---|---|---|
| Warm-up | Gentle callisthenics (free standing exercises) to include stretching exercises. Walking, jogging or running on the spot could be included. | 5–10 minutes |
| Aerobic exercise | Continuous brisk/fast walking, jogging, running, cycling, swimming, circuit training or dancing. | 20-plus minutes |
| Muscle conditioning | Strengthening exercises using actual body weight, free weights or weight machines. | 5–10 minutes |
| Warm-down | Gentle stretching, then relaxing exercises. | 5 minutes |

Notes

i. If required there could be a short recovery period between the aerobic and muscle conditioning phases.

ii. If preferred, the muscle conditioning phase could precede the aerobic phase, though recent research at California State University found that this arrangement can make the workout harder.

## When to Exercise

The time of day when you take exercise can be relevant to the effectiveness of training. If you exercise before meal times it will have a depressive effect on the appetite; therefore you will not normally feel hungry after a fairly intensive exercise session. If the exercise taken has been sufficiently vigorous it will ensure an 'after burn' effect, whereby the body will continue to burn up additional calories well after the training period has actually ceased. Both phenomena can assist with weight control.

Light exercise such as a gentle walk taken after a meal will assist the movement of food through the intestines and help digestion. Vigorous exercise should not be performed soon after a meal, for the large amount of blood that will have flowed to the abdomen to assist the digestion and absorption of food will be diverted to the working muscles. This could interrupt the natural process of digestion and cause discomfort.

The efficiency of our body is controlled by the periodic release throughout the day of hormones such as thyroxine and other thyroid hormones from the thyroid gland (which controls levels of activity); adrenalin from the adrenal gland (which raises the heartbeat and blood pressure); and cortisol, also from the adrenal gland (released in stress). The release of these chemicals has a wide-reaching influence on the body's daily physical and mental performance. For example, peak levels of cortisol are achieved soon after we wake up, which ensures that our short-term memory is at its best at this time of day – a good time to make mental notes of what to do later.

The surge of adrenalin that accompanies our waking can stimulate athletic 'freaks' to leap out of bed and go for a run. For those who do so, it is of great importance that they carry out a progressive warm-up first before exerting themselves. However, if you are over 40 or older, it is not a good idea to participate in exercise or activity that is of such a strenuous nature at this time of day. The heart muscle can be sensitive to sudden exertion up to about two hours after getting out of bed and it is a time when the body is more prone to heart attacks. It is therefore best for these people to pace themselves first thing in the morning. Though many asthmatics can now take part safely in regular exercising, research at John Moore's University, Liverpool, has found that chest tightening is often greater in the early morning despite the effects of medication. It is therefore advisable for asthmatics to exercise later in the day.

The midday/early afternoon period is an ideal time for a break – the traditional siesta – because this is the time of day when the body's glucose levels drop and changes in hormone levels can make concentrated work more difficult. The late afternoon is when motor skills can best be learnt and practised, whether it be golf or DIY. It is believed that the heart is at its most efficient in the early evening, making it the ideal time for exercise and for taking part in sports that require strength or endurance. If it is possible to follow this hormonal clock then perhaps it can be to our advantage.

## Warming Up and Warming Down

Like any machine the human body functions more efficiently, and is less likely to suffer damage, if it is warmed up before It is called upon the meet the demands of stress. The most effective types of warm-up are those activities that increase the heart rate; the rate and depth of breathing; and blood and muscle temperature. The warm-up also ensures that the blood pressure is raised, blood is diverted to the working muscles and that the body, as a total entity, is given the opportunity to mobilise its resources to meet the demands of overload or exercise stress. It also prepares you mentally to anticipate the demands of sustained effort.

In cold weather the warm-up is essential for, in order to reduce heat loss in these conditions, the body shuts down many blood vessels and the workload on the heart is increased. You should wrap up well with extra clothing, plus perhaps a woollen hat and mitts, to help get the body temperature well up and the blood circulating before you commence any hard exercise.

A warm-up can take a variety of forms, from running on the spot to brisk walking or slow jogging, all combined with simple low intensity callisthenics. Whenever possible the warm-up should relate to the specific form of exercise to follow. So after an initial warm-up, if the activity to follow is to be squash or tennis, continue by swinging the arms to simulate racket drives. Similarly, simulated discus throws or golf swings will help prepare the muscles and joints for those activities. If you are going to swim, gently stretch the muscles and joints of the shoulders with loosening exercises, then simulate crawl or breaststroke. If you are going to run you need to prepare the legs, so gently stretch the muscles and tendons of your thighs, calves and instep.

The conclusion of an exercise session is important, for a systematic warming-down increases the effectiveness of the training. Don't end your exercise session suddenly. A gradual reduction in the intensity of the activity over a few minutes helps the circulation to remove waste products that are a result of exercise. Post-exercise stiffness and any possible loss of suppleness can also be avoided by carrying out stretching and loosening exercises. This is particularly important after jogging or cycling some distance. The warming-down phase of training should therefore be an integral part of your exercise programme.

Basic exercises suitable for a general warm-up and warm-down are to be found under level 1 of the home exercise callisthenic exercises shown in chapter 10. Warming-up and warming-down exercises that include stretching exercises, which are suitable for the more athletic, are shown in figure 35 on page 145.

## Rest and Recovery

The body requires time to recover from the demands imposed upon it in each exercise session. Recovery periods should be regarded as important as the time spent exercising: this is the time when the beneficial physiological adaptations stimulated by exercise take place and the training effect occurs. Recovery time can be taken as periods of passive rest with little activity, or as active rest involving light exercise, massage and gentle stretching. Active rest stimulates the circulatory system, ensuring the removal of waste products and resupply of muscles, organs and tissue with oxygen and nutrients.

The concept of exercising every other day three times a week ensures that the body can adapt and recover during the resting periods. An effective exercise programme must comprise a controlled balance of physical effort and recovery. If the balance is correct a steady improvement in fitness will follow. But if the exercise stress is great, and insufficient time is allowed to replace the body's energy stores and remove waste products, fitness will in fact deteriorate.

Constant moderate exercise, even of a comparatively low intensity such as brisk walking, produces a feeling of well-being and also has a tranquillising effect upon the nervous system. More vigorous exercise of a high aerobic nature can give a euphoric feeling, accompanied by the sensation of exhilaration, calmness and unlimited energy. These sensations are sometimes referred to as a 'runner's high' and are caused by the release into the blood of chemicals known as endorphins that have a mood-elevating effect.

Excess exercise can result in a greater release of chemicals into the system. Some leisure-time exercisers go to the unwise extremes of working out for two or three hours a day. The result is that they become addicted to further exercise by the mood-elevating endorphin chemicals in the brain and will not stop exercising, even when injured and suffering pain. If they are forced to stop exercising, whatever the reason, these exercise addicts can experience unpleasant symptoms similar to drug withdrawal cases – loss of appetite, depression, restlessness and sleeplessness.

It is believed that exercise may enhance the body's immune system by regulating the release of hormones and chemicals into the bloodstream, so warding off infection and also alleviating stress. It is also thought that moderate exercise may help counter the decrease in immune response associated with ageing. However, regular exhaustive exercise can be stressful to the body, even to the extent of damaging a person's immune response. In these circumstances the degree of damage would depend on the health of each individual and the intensity of the exercise. It is possible to over-exercise through not allowing sufficient recovery time between training sessions. This can occur at all levels of fitness. It usually results from the gradual build-up of the effects of fairly hard training sessions, followed by insufficient rest periods, and not as a result of very hard individual training sessions.

The common symptoms of over-training can be identified as follows:

a. Lack of energy.
b. An increase in basal pulse rate (to be taken before you get out of bed).
c. Excessive fatigue after a normal workout.
d. Unusual irritability.
e. Difficulty in getting to sleep, or waking up early.
f. Increase in infections resulting in sore throat, colds, sore lips etc.
g. Dizziness experienced when standing up quickly.
h. Miscellaneous aches and pains.
i. Lack of enthusiasm for exercise and lack of progress in training.

Always listen to what your body has to tell you. If you are constantly experiencing one or more of the above symptoms you could be over-exercising, so take a rest of two days or more, relax, have hot baths, perhaps a sauna and massage. When you recommence training reduce the intensity initially. If the symptoms reoccur, transfer to a less taxing programme or activity. Should you also experience any of the symptoms outlined below under the heading Medical Precautions, you should immediately stop exercising and see your doctor.

From time to time it may not be possible to continue your training programme for a period, perhaps due to injury, family commitments, the need to travel, or work duties. Not being able to exercise can be disappointing and frustrating, particularly after the time it may have taken to get fit. Don't despair. Though your degree of aerobic fitness will fall quickly by about 30 per cent in a matter of two weeks or so, even if you cannot do any exercise you should retain 50–70 per cent of your endurance for three months or more.

## A Fitness Diary/Log

A fitness diary or log is an excellent training aid. Dependent on the type of activities pursued, it is possible to record a variety of detail, such as performance planned and actually achieved in distance; time; speed; together with comment as to how you feel on the day and weather and wind conditions. You can also record incidents, injuries, terrain and ground conditions underfoot, and details of circuit training or weight training undertaken. Keeping a diary gives a stimulus to goals to be aimed for and achieved. Details of an exercise log and various training cards are found on pages 64, 74, 106, 119 and 226.

Details of an exercise log and various training cards are found on pages 64, 74, 106, 119 and 226.

### MEDICAL PRECAUTIONS

If you have any reason to doubt your medical condition before you embark on any exercise programme, it is wise to consider the need for a medical check. If you are overweight; are aged over 40; are grossly unfit; have a medical disorder that requires that you take medicine or treatment (for high blood pressure, diabetes, arthritis etc.); or if you have any other reason to doubt your medical condition, you should get yourself checked out by your physician *before you undertake any level of physical activity to which you are unaccustomed.*

If when exercising you develop chest pain, dizziness or severe headache; feel sick; experience unusual excessive fatigue, more than usual shortness of breath, pain and discomfort or difficulty in moving parts of the body; experience abnormal nerve sensations; or become unco-ordinated and cannot move in a straight line, you should *immediately* stop exercising and, *as soon as possible*, see your physician.

Don't exercise if you have a heavy cold, the flu or are otherwise feeling unwell. Avoid exercising in extremely hot weather, when the humidity is over 60 per cent, or if the conditions are extremely cold. Remember that recreational exercise should be enjoyable.

As one eminent doctor is reported to have advised his

patient, 'You don't have to go out and kill yourself to improve your health. Just get a good pair of walking shoes and enjoy life. Come back and see me when you've worn them out.'

## EXERCISE TIPS

1. Well-fitting, cushioned footwear with a good grip give stability and reduce the possibility of lower leg and back injuries – particularly so with activities like running, hopping and skipping. If necessary, seek advice from your local specialist sports retailer so that what you wear is suitable for the activities planned.

2. When taking part in aerobic-type movements (see page 227), particularly those that involve high impact exercise, the floor surface should be shock absorbing. Sprung wooden floors, carpet laid on suitable padding over a hard surface, or gymnastic mats absorb impact well (though gymnastic mats can lack stability). Asphalt and concrete have poor impact absorption but offer good stability control and friction grip, suitable for short sprints and minor games; but well-cushioned footwear should be worn.

3. Do not push yourself too hard as you build up fitness.

4. Always have a rest day between exercise sessions.

5. Do not exercise after a heavy meal or after drinking alcohol.

6. Drink plenty of water. Water keeps the body systems working efficiently. Unlike other fluids, water has the unique quality that enables it to be absorbed quickly into the body.
When we exercise, the muscles produce extra heat that must be expelled to keep the body working properly, so fluid is given off in perspiration and water vapour breathed out. This amount of fluid is increased if clothes do not 'breathe' properly and allow perspiration to evaporate. The harder and longer exercise takes place and the hotter and more humid the atmosphere, the more fluid is lost from the body. During an

hour of general exercise about a litre (1¾ pints) of fluid can be lost. Running or brisk cycling for the same time can double that amount. If exercise is prolonged without replenishment of the fluid lost, the exerciser will suffer dehydration, a condition that can affect both performance and health.

Take note that thirst is a poor indicator of the body's condition. If you feel thirsty at any point before or during an exercise session, you are already becoming dehydrated. As with most problems, prevention is better than cure. Drink water before and during a workout and, after exercising, perhaps unsweetened fruit juice diluted with water with a pinch of sea salt to help replace the body minerals given off in perspiration. Sports drinks are relatively new to the exercise market. They are popular and pleasant tasting, but do little that water, fruit juice and some added salt cannot do.

7. Cold weather should not serve as a deterrent to the physically fit, provided that the conditions are not extreme and safeguards are taken – such as the wearing of suitable clothing and footwear. Also wear a close-knit scarf over the nose and mouth to help warm the air taken into the lungs. This ensures that the windpipe is kept warm and that the body is not chilled internally from the effects of cold air breathed in that could place an added strain on the heart. Those who are not fit should really avoid exercising in such conditions.

8. If for some reason you cannot keep up your exercise programme and are unable to exercise for a week or more, when recommencing, restart at a lower level of intensity than you were at when you laid off. This could be only half or two-thirds of what you were doing previously. If you had to stop exercising because of an illness, make sure that you are totally recovered before recommencing and restart at a very much lower intensity. Only attempt any progressions when you are ready to do so. After a serious illness, or any illness that may have affected the heart and lungs, it is wise to have a medical examination before restarting an exercise programme.

9. Should an injury be sustained while exercising, if the injury is severe or gives concern, see a doctor. More minor exercise-

Figure 7: Exercise Log

| DATE | EXERCISE | INTENSITY | DURATION/ DISTANCE | COMMENTS |
|------|----------|-----------|--------------------|----------|
| 1.7.97 | Walking | Brisk 3 m.p.h. | 2 hours/ 6 miles | Moorland track. Dry, warm conditions. |
| 3.7.97 | Weight training (8 exercises) | 3 sets of 10 reps | — | Now need to increase reps slightly. |
| 5.7.97 | Cycling | Moderate pace | 1 hour/ 12 miles | Into slight breeze on canal towpath. |
| 7.7.97 | Swimming | Comfortable pace | 6 lengths/ x 50 metres | Breaststroke and backstroke (untimed). Could increase lengths, perhaps by two. |

related injuries may require you to stop exercising. A cold compress, ice pack or packet of frozen peas suitably wrapped in a towel or cloth to avoid contact with the skin, together with an elasticated bandage wrapped directly around the area with the part elevated, can help keep swelling to a minimum. If necessary seek medical advice. This could speed recovery through expert rehabilitation treatment, perhaps with the application of heat or massage, or by mobilising the area.

# FIVE

# Exercising for Stamina

- Aerobic Fitness Requirements
- Walking
    Benefits
    Programme Aims
    Progressive Walking Exercises
- Running
    Jogging
    Interval Running
    Fartlek Running
- Cycling
    Equipment
    Basic Cycling Technique
    Progressive Training
- Swimming
    Overcoming Difficulties
- Circuit Training
    Inital Testing
    Trim Trails

Stamina is the main ingredient of general fitness. The degree of stamina we possess depends as much on the efficiency of the heart and lungs as on the working muscles. Stamina, or endurance fitness, is the cornerstone on which all forms of fitness can be built. It can be achieved in a variety of ways – through sport, walking, swimming, forms of running such as jogging, fartlek and interval running, or circuit training. Exercise that aims to improve stamina – including training for the core activities of walking, running, cycling and swimming

– falls into the category of aerobic exercise. The techniques, training principles and progressions for these activities are outlined in this chapter, preceded by an analysis of the aerobic fitness values of popular activities and games. Note that many of the programmes that follow are described in the conventional measurement of miles, yards and feet for clarity as to stride length, distance and speed. The various programmes outlined in this chapter are suitable for a wide range of ability but are particularly suited for individuals with a low aerobic capacity.

## AEROBIC FITNESS REQUIREMENTS — ACTIVITIES AND GAMES

The aerobic capacity required to carry out different activities and games varies considerably. Certain activities such as circuit training call for a continuous oxygen intake and a sound degree of cardiovascular fitness so as to tolerate the ongoing demands of the high intensity exercise. Others, like the sport of cricket, are more sedentary but still have some degree of aerobic value, though of a lesser nature. The table in figure 8 lists a variety of activities and sports and gives their respective aerobic values in general terms. It can be seen that the core fitness activities of walking, running, swimming and cycling score highly on the four-point scale (four being the highest), as do rowing, squash, circuit training and cross-country skiing. The major sports of soccer, rugby and hockey equate equally. Gardening (digging and raking) have established values, whereas golf and cricket are at the lower end of the scale having periods of non-activity. Note that the table should be used only as a rough guide as a great deal will depend on the effort put into the activity.

Figure 8: Aerobic Values of Activities and Games

| ACTIVITY | AEROBIC VALUE | ACTIVITY | AEROBIC VALUE |
|---|---|---|---|
| Badminton | 2 | Jogging | 3 |
| Basketball | 3 | Netball | 2 |
| Callisthenics (vigorous) | 3 | Orienteering | 2–3 |
| Canoeing (competitive long distance | 3–4 | Rowing | 4 |
| | | Rugby | 2–3 |
| Canoeing (recreational) | 1–2 | Running (distance) | 4 |
| Circuit training | 3–4 | Shooting (rough) | 1–2 |
| Climbing stairs (continuous) | 3–4 | Skiing (cross-country) | 4 |
| Cricket | 1 | Skiing (downhill) | 2 |
| Cycling (hard continuous) | 4 | Skipping (continuous) | 2–3 |
| Dancing (vigorous aerobic) | 3 | Squash | 3–4 |
| Football | 2–3 | Swimming (competitive) | 4 |
| Gardening (continuous digging and raking) | 2 | Swimming (recreational) | 1–2 |
| | | Tennis | 2–3 |
| Golf | 1–2 | Volleyball | 2–3 |
| Handball | 3 | Walking (brisk) | 2–3 |
| Hockey | 2–3 | Walking (fast) | 3–4 |
| Horse-riding (recreational) | 1 | Weight training | 2–3 |
| Housework | 1 | | |

## WALKING

BENEFITS

Walking is an excellent form of aerobic exercise. Due to the structure of our musculo-skeletal system and the curvature and flexibility of the spine, it is the most natural exercise for the human body. It is also a form of exercise that has low risk of injury and requires no special clothing, equipment, or prepared training area. Carried out correctly, it has beneficial effects on posture and is helpful to weight reduction. Walking can be done on your own or in company and, within reason, in most weather provided you wear suitable apparel. It helps to reduce stress and tension while giving a definite feeling of well-being. Walking gives you time to think and time to drink in the surroundings. It is a cost-free form of therapy, a unique form of exercise in that it is safe to perform and can make for longevity.

## Footwear

It is not necessary to obtain any custom-made shoes for normal walking, but what you wear must be comfortable and, according to the surface of the ground, safe to use. The uppers should be soft and flexible so as to bend with the movement of the foot. The sole should be strong, flexible, non-slip and also thick enough to protect the feet from stones or rough surfaces. Synthetic material should be avoided because the material does not breathe, can cause the feet to perspire and even become slippery. Shoes with a heel of about an inch or just over are best as they avoid any tension on the Achilles tendon, whereas low heels can, after a while, exert a painful pull on the tendon. A high heel can be unstable and unbalance the body on uneven surfaces, leading possibly to a twisted ankle. If you are considering walking on rough ground or over hill country then walking boots are essential, for they will give support to the ankles.

## Walking Technique

When you walk, keep your shoulders back and pull your tummy in. Walk with a smooth, effortless, comfortable stride, aiming to develop an easy rhythm. Point your feet straight forward, the heel of the leading foot touching the ground with the lead leg fully but not over extended. Then roll on to the ball of the foot, after which push off the toes. The arms should swing naturally to balance the body.

### PROGRAMME AIMS

The aims of any walking programme should be two-fold. Firstly, to obtain the aerobic benefits that this enjoyable exercise offers. Secondly, to develop and maintain good posture.

First of all, select an area of level ground and allow the body to become accustomed to the exercise without any undue strain on joints and muscles. The pace you walk at will depend on your standard of fitness, age and ability. If, when you start, you are soon out of breath then you are walking too fast and need to slow down. If necessary, stop and have a short rest before carrying on at a slower pace. You should be familiar with the area you are walking so that easily identified and pre-measured checkpoints will help confirm the distance you have covered in a set time.

## Starter Programmes

If you are not used to walking it is best to adhere to a starter programme. Two programmes are given, both based on progressing from an initial 15-minute walking exercise session.

PROGRAMME I **(figure 9)** This is a simple programme for the unaccustomed walker, with easy progressions. First of all, after a warm-up, see how far you can walk in 15 minutes at a comfortable continuous pace. Having noted the distance and exercising every other day, continue exercising at the same pace but divide the time in half so that you walk out for the first half of seven and a half minutes, then back to the start point in the second half of the exercise session. After about two weeks, or when you feel ready, add two minutes to the total time, one minute walking out and one minute back. Repeat this progression by adding a further

Figure 9: Starter Walking Programme I

| STAGE | TIMES WEEKLY | WALKING TIME |
|---|---|---|
| *Initial test* | | 15 minutes |
| 1 | 3–4 | 7½ minutes out, 7½ minutes back |
| 2 | 3–4 | 8½ minutes out, 8½ minutes back |
| 3 | 3–4 | 9½ minutes out, 9½ minutes back |
| 4 | 3–4 | 10½ minutes out, 10½ minutes back |
| *Retest* | | 15 minutes |

two minutes every two weeks or when you are ready. As you build up the distance you should now be able to walk faster. After exercising perhaps for one month, check the improvement in your pace by walking for 15 minutes and compare the distance now walked with the distance you originally covered in the same time. Further progressions can be made by adding four minutes each fortnight or so, also by walking up modest gradients.

PROGRAMME 2 (figure 10) In this programme the progressive exercise times advance 15 minutes at each stage. First of all, after a warm-up, see how far you can walk at a comfortable continuous pace in 15 minutes to assess which pace category you fall into – slow (2 mph), brisk (3 mph) or fast (4 mph). Having identified your pace commence walking every other day at the same pace (stage 1). In the second week of the starter programme, or when you are ready, the plan will be to increase your walking time to 30 minutes (stage 2), again walking every other day at the same pace as the first week.

In the third week, or when you are ready, the walking time is increased to 45 minutes (stage 3) and in the fourth week to one hour (stage 4), all at the same pace – i.e. slow, brisk or fast. Variations can be made to this starter programme, though it is important the progressions do not impose discomfort or strain. You may feel that because your basic standard of walking fitness is found to be improving rapidly, you wish to increase your pace rather than continue the slow pace programme throughout the four-week/stage period, gradually moving up from a half-mile in 15 minutes to two miles in 60 minutes. For example, you could, after following the slow pace programme for the first two weeks/stages, transfer across to the brisk pace over one and a half miles in 30 minutes on your third week/stage and a brisk pace two and a quarter miles in 45 minutes in the fourth week/stage. But any progress should not impose an undue strain on the heart and lungs, nor on the muscles and tendons. If you find that you are out of breath and cannot talk while walking, you are going too fast, so *slow down*. If the breathless symptoms persist, or any other unusual symptoms occur, it is wise to see your doctor.

Figure 10: Starter Walking Programme 2

| WEEK/ STAGE | TIMES WEEKLY | WALKING TIME (MINUTES) | SLOW PACE 2 MPH (MILES) | BRISK PACE 3 MPH (MILES) | FAST PACE 4 MPH (MILES) |
|---|---|---|---|---|---|
| 1 | 3–4 | 15 | ½ | ¾ | 1 |
| 2 | 3–4 | 30 | 1 | 1½ | 2 |
| 3 | 3–4 | 45 | 1½ | 2¼ | |
| 4 | 3–4 | 60 | 2 | 3 | 4 |

## Speed and Distance

An appreciation of the time it takes to walk a mile at slow, brisk and fast pace will help in the planning and enjoyment of your walks. A mile at 2 mph will take 30 minutes, at 3 mph 20 minutes and at 4 mph 15 minutes, though this latter pace is normally too fast for many people to keep up. Figure 11 is a useful guide to the time it takes to cover distance from half a mile to four miles.

Figure 11: Walking – Time, Distance and Pace

| DISTANCE (MILES) | SLOW PACE 2 MPH (MINUTES) | BRISK PACE 3 MPH (MINUTES) | FAST PACE 4 MPH (MINUTES) |
|---|---|---|---|
| ½ | 15 | 10 | 7½ |
| 1 | 30 | 20 | 15 |
| 1½ | 45 | 30 | 22½ |
| 2 | 60 | 40 | 30 |
| 2½ | 75 | 50 | 37½ |
| 3 | 90 | 60 | 45 |
| 3½ | 105 | 70 | 52½ |
| 4 | 120 | 80 | 60 |

Figure 12: How to Measure Stride Length

**Walk, jog or run ten steps. Measure the distance travelled in feet and divide by ten.**

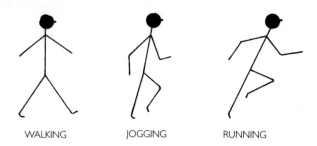

WALKING          JOGGING          RUNNING

Figure 13: How to Use a Pedometer

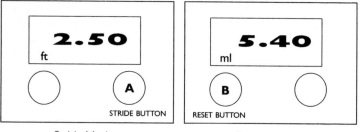

Stride Mode          Distance Mode

1. A typical electronic pedometer, to be worn on the belt, has a large electronic display with inputs for stride length (one to six feet) and for distance (up to 999.99 miles).
2. To set the pedometer press stride button A to record the stride length required. Each press increases the stride by 0.1 feet until the stride required is shown, here recorded in figure 13A as 2.50 ft. After five seconds the FT (stride mode) will revert to ML (distance mode).
3. Figure 13B shows the display in distance mode recording 5.40 miles covered.
4. Pressing the reset button B will clear the screen of any distance already recorded.

It is useful to be able to judge the distance covered according to your stride length and pace. One way is to measure your stride (figure 12), which may be between two and three and a half feet, and use a watch. As there are 5,280 feet to the mile, if your average stride is two feet it will take 2,640 strides to cover the mile. As you walk, glance at the sweep of the second hand of your watch and count the number of paces you take in ten seconds. Supposing it is 22, you then multiply that by six to give the number of paces taken in one minute; this comes to 132 paces, which divided into 2,640 gives 20, that is a mile in 20 minutes – a walking speed of about 3 mph. Figure 14 gives details of various stride-lengths relating to pace and time.

Figure 14: Walking – Stride, Pace and Time

| | STEPS PER MINUTE (STEPS PER 10 SECONDS) | | | | |
|---|---|---|---|---|---|
| APPROX. MILES PER HOUR | 2FT STRIDE | 2½FT STRIDE | 3FT STRIDE | 3½FT STRIDE | APPROX. MINS PER MILE |
| 2 | 90 (15) | 66 (11) | 60 (10) | 54 (9) | 30 |
| 2½ | 108 (18) | 90 (15) | 72 (12) | 66 (11) | 24 |
| 3 | 132 (22) | 102 (17) | 90 (15) | 78 (13) | 20 |
| 3½ | 156 (26) | 120 (20) | 102 (17) | 96 (16) | 17 |
| 4 | 174 (29) | 138(23) | 120 (20) | 102 (17) | 15 |
| 4½ | 198 (33) | 156 (26) | 132 (22) | 120 (20) | 13 |
| 5 | 216 (36) | 174 (29) | 144 (24) | 132 (22) | 12 |
| 5½ | – | – | 156 (26) | 144 (24) | 11 |
| | | NOMINAL STRIDES PER MILE | | | |
| | 2,640 | 2,112 | 1, 760 | 1, 624 | |

Another way to check distance is to use a pedometer, obtainable from sports shops (see figure 13). This resembles a watch. Once the instrument is adjusted to your average stride length and strapped to your belt, the action of walking will cause the pedometer to oscillate and trigger its mechanism to register the distance covered. It is possible to purchase a jog-and-walk watch which, in addition to acting as a pedometer with walking and jogging modes, is also a stopwatch.

A third way to judge distance and time is to be completely familiar with your walking course so that mile and half-mile points are well known to you (perhaps verified by previous checks with a car or cycle mileometer, or by careful study of a suitably scaled map).

Once you have completed either starter programme, you should be able to pursue a half-hour or one-hour progressive programme respectively, exercising every other day. Gradually increase the length of your walks, but practise over the increased distance several times before you walk any further. Remember, whatever pace you select, you must feel comfortable. Set out well-defined goals and keep interesting records of your walks as indicated on a walking record card (see figure 15). The regularity and consistency of your programme is significant, as is the time taken on your walk for, dependent on your weight, when walking at a brisk pace you can burn off about 150 to 200 calories for every 30 minutes of fitness walking.

Figure 15: Walking Record Card

| DATE | FROM | TO | MILES | PACE | TIME | M.P.H. | COMMENTS |
|---|---|---|---|---|---|---|---|
| 1.3.98 | Pickwick | Broughton Via Neston | 6 | Brisk | 2 hrs | 3 | Undulating lanes. Still, dry, sunny day |
| 3.3.98 | Broughton | Melsham and back | 4 | Fast | 1 hr | 4 | Flat walk. Still, dry day |
| 5.3.98 | Bradford on Avon | Semington | 5 | Fast | 1 hr 15 mins | 4 | Headwind on towpath. A harder but satisfying walk |
| 7.3.98 | Bathampton | Bradford on Avon | 8 | Brisk | 2 hrs 40 mins | 3 | Towpath walk. Wet conditions into breeze. |
| Weekly Totals | | | 23 | | 6 hrs 55 mins | | |

Pace Variation

As with other forms of exercise, it is possible to apply the principle of overload to walking by exercising regularly against an increasing task – for instance duration or pace, so that one can eventually walk further or faster. Here are some examples that can be introduced into your personal walking programme.

INCREASING PACE The example below shows how the gradual application of the principle of overload can help a fit but slow walker, exercising every other day, move up to a brisk pace.

  a. Walk for 25 minutes at a slow pace, then for a further five minutes at a brisk pace. Repeat the exercise every two days for four exercise sessions.
  b. Walk for 20 minutes at a slow pace, then for a further ten minutes at a brisk pace. Repeat the exercise every two days for four exercise sessions.
  c. Repeat as above, every four days gradually decreasing the slow pace element and increasing the brisk pace element until you walk for the whole 30 minutes at brisk pace.

THE 15-MINUTE MILE Four mph, or a mile in 15 minutes, is a very good walking pace and, for some, a desirable goal. A sensible way to build up to this target is to progress through the following stages According to your personal fitness standard, practise the schedule every other day, repeating each standard four times. Or move to the next standard when you are ready.

  a. Walk for 15 minutes at a brisk pace.
  b. Walk for ten minutes at a brisk pace, then a further five at a fast pace.
  c. Walk for five minutes at a brisk pace, then ten minutes at a fast pace.
  d. Walk for 15 minutes at a fast pace. You have cracked it!

Once the 15-minute mile has been achieved you may wish to build up gradually, using the same principles, to cover two miles in 30 minutes. When this is comfortably achieved, three miles in 45 minutes may be possible and eventually four miles in an hour. But don't try to increase your speed over a distance before you are ready to do so.

Other Variations

A variation in pace can be made by carrying out periods of brisk walking for a set time interspersed with moving up a gear to a fast walk. It is best not to make a walk a speed or endurance test. Enjoy your walk, for what you see along the way is as important as how far you travel.

SCOUT PACE This consists of trotting for a set number of paces, perhaps 30 to 50, then walking a number of paces before trotting again. The young and athletic can cover a mile in ten to twelve minutes, or even less, in this fashion without undue fatigue. You can, if you wish, adapt the scout pace to give an interesting variation to your walk by introducing a gentle light jog perhaps of just 20 to 40 paces every so many 100 yards. The jog can be gradually increased over several walks to, say, 100 paces applied every 400 or 500 yards or more. Such variations on a long walk can serve to relieve pressure points on the feet and help circulation. However, remember to jog lightly. The impact force of the feet hitting the ground when you are running can be over double your body weight at each stride. Also, you should seek to avoid breathlessness.

HILLS AND SLOPES Other variations in pace can be applied on undulating terrain. It is possible to speed up on a slight downhill slope. When going uphill, reduce your stride but if you can, keep up the same pace even though you are ascending.

DISTANCE WALKING When planning a long walk select a steady, comfortable, constant pace that can be maintained indefinitely with a good rhythm. On a long walk of several hours, have frequent drinks and rest for a few minutes each hour. If possible, relax completely with your feet up on a log, rock or rucksack so that the blood that has collected in your legs and feet will drain away; but avoid resting too long, as your back and leg muscles will stiffen. Before you set off again have a gentle loosen up.

POWER WALKING This is a dynamic approach to walking and is becoming increasingly popular with keep-fit classes and aerobic-type sessions. It involves a determined, fast stride with an accompanying exaggerated high, bent arm pumping action and can be accompanied by the use of light hand weights to assist the upper body muscle tone. These hand weights fit comfortably into the palm of the hand, with an elasticated supporting strap that runs across the back of the hand, and weigh about 450 g. Power walking can be carried out in a suitable indoor area, the walker describing circles or figure-of-eight patterns, or outdoors over a distance. The whole action requires greater energy and effort than normal walking technique. Power walking is fun but the technique is not suitable if you are going to walk any distance that requires conservation of energy to achieve your aim.

In conclusion it must be said that when analysing energy used and fat lost, the effects of sustained exercise are more important than the effects of high intensity exercise carried out over a short period. Walking at the brisk pace of 3 mph for 15 minutes uses over ten times the amount of energy expended in 40 press-ups, even though press-ups can be an exhausting exercise to perform. It is therefore not necessary to puff and perspire profusely to burn calories. Walking at a brisk pace is an excellent exercise.

Walking is fun, whether you add some walking to your journey to work, or walk in the lunchtime work-break. At other times you can explore the parks in your region or take a bus ride into the country where you will find bridleways and footpaths. If you wish for company and people of similar interests, there are rambling clubs to join. There are also many national footpaths to follow that include Offa's Dyke, Pembrokeshire Coastal Path, the Pennine Way, Cleveland Way, North Downs Way, South Downs Way, Ridgeway Path, South West Coastal Path and West Highland Way. If you are very fit, venturesome, adequately trained and equipped, the Roof of Wales walk will take you from the Roman Road, the Sarn Helen north of Neath, across the Brecons, the Cambrian mountains and then Plynlimon to North Wales. It is a trek that I found memorable in its scenery, wildlife and soul-searching solitude. But above all walking can be for the family and will last a lifetime.

## RUNNING

Running is a simple, natural, convenient and practical way of improving and maintaining stamina. It requires minimum equipment and facilities and can take various forms including jogging, 'fartlek' (speed play) and interval running. Whatever form of running you undertake, it can be fun, free and a quick way to get fit.

### Footwear

A good pair of training shoes is the only equipment you will need. They must be comfortable when worn with athletic socks, allowing the toes room to be wriggled. Your heel must not slide about, though not be held so tightly as to cause blisters. The collar is best cushioned, the insole soft and yielding to take any shock and give good arch support. The heel should be high enough to avoid strain on the Achilles tendon and calves. The sole must be even and layered to lessen impact and thick enough to protect from stones and flints underfoot. The sole should also have some flexibility and bend in the hands. It must have a good tread, so as to give traction on slippery surfaces, and can be slightly swept up at the toe and heel to allow a smooth running action. Training shoes are best bought in the late afternoon in order to get a good fit, for if you have been walking about for some time, your feet will have swollen a little and the size selected must not pinch at any time. A well-fitting training shoe ensures not only your comfort, but helps avoid minor injuries.

### JOGGING

Jogging can be looked upon as running for beginners, but also as a serious exercise in its own right. The main difference between running and jogging is that of pace. If you can cover a mile in less than eight minutes you are running, if slower you are jogging. Jogging is not a suitable exercise for those considerably overweight, or who have suffered injuries or arthritis of the hips, back or legs. They might try swimming or cycling instead. Elderly people should avoid jogging, though there are some notable elderly long-distance runners – however, these people are exceptions and have been running for most of their lives.

### Jogging Technique

When you commence to jog, your body should be relaxed, erect, and with the head up. Elbows should be bent at 90°, the arms swung easily in rhythm with your leg action, hands also relaxed. The heel of the leading foot should strike the ground lightly, without over-striding, then roll smoothly over on to the ball of the foot. The whole action should be natural and comfortable.

### A Beginner's Training Course and Programme

A beginner's programme can be based on a training course of pre-set distances to be walked or jogged. These distances are best marked as exercise units on the course that may comprise a running track, sports field or open ground. Quiet lanes and roads may be suitable too. Street lamps and telegraph poles are normally spaced about 50 yards apart and that is the distance which will serve as a training unit in the exercise described. Figure 16 gives an example of the plan of a beginner's jogging course using local features (or flags or sticks) to make up the 50-yard units. If it is not possible to train on the marked course or use street lamps or telegraph poles as markers, you can count your walking and jogging paces, so ensuring a similar constant measure of distance covered.

Following a general warm-up each exercise session should last for 15 minutes, when you would jog and walk according to your ability. For example, a beginner who has not done much exercise for some time would start by walking four units then jogging one, followed by walking four units then again jogging one unit, and so on. His/her aim is gradually to reduce the walking and increase the jogging phases until he/she is jogging continuously for the 15-minute exercise period.

## Guiding Principles

There can be no set programme that will suit beginners of different ages and abilities and also those who have not done any exercise for some time. However, the following training principles apply to all abilities. Firstly, progressions should be gentle, with the aim of cutting down the amount of walking and increasing the jogging element, until after a while – whether this is days, weeks or even longer – you are capable of jogging continuously for 15 minutes. Secondly, if at any stage your state of breathing is such that you are not able to carry out a conversation with a jogging partner (real or imaginary), you could be doing too much, so stop jogging and start walking!

Figure 16: Beginner's Jogging Course

THIS DIAGRAM SHOWS HOW NATURAL FEATURES CAN BE USED AS 50-YARD/METRE UNITS. THE AIM IS TO REDUCE THE AMOUNT OF WALKING AND INCREASE THE AMOUNT OF JOGGING (SEE TEXT).

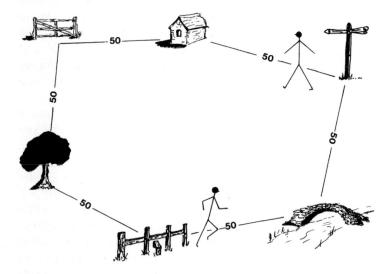

Figure 17: Beginner's Walking/Jogging Programme

| STAGE | | | | | | | | | | | | | |
|---|---|---|---|---|---|---|---|---|---|---|---|---|---|
| 1 | W | W | W | W | J | W | W | W | W | J | W | W | W |
| 2 | W | W | W | W | J | J | W | W | W | W | J | J | W |
| 3 | W | W | W | J | J | W | W | W | J | J | W | W | W |
| 4 | W | W | W | J | J | J | W | W | W | J | J | J | W |
| 5 | W | W | J | J | J | W | W | J | J | J | W | W | J |
| 6 | W | W | J | J | J | J | W | W | J | J | J | J | W |
| 7 | W | J | J | J | J | W | J | J | J | J | W | J | J |
| 8 | J | J | J | J | J | J | J | J | J | J | J | J | J |

<50> yards

Key W = Walk J = Jog

REPEAT PATTERN FOR TOTAL TIME OF 15 MINUTES

## Variations to the Beginner's Programme

In the programme shown in figure 17 a beginner, who is a little less capable than that previously mentioned, first walks a greater number of units. The example shown gives four units of walking (4 x 50 yards = 200 yards), followed by a 50-yard jog. Older or less fit people may be more comfortable initially walking further, perhaps seven units (350 yards or more), before jogging one unit. The walking/jogging sequence is then repeated throughout the 15-minute exercise session. As the person becomes fitter, the walking element is reduced at each stage as he/she progresses and the jogging element gradually increased until he/she is capable of jogging the whole 15 minutes.

Further progressions can be achieved by gradually increasing your jogging speed and the distance covered per session. The unit jogging programme can be adapted further for use by the older or heavier person. Benefit can be obtained by walking a distance, say, 300 yards (or paces), and then jogging, but only for 25–30 yards (or paces); and repeating this sequence throughout the session. The jogging phase would then be gradually, though minimally, built up and the walking phase similarly decreased without imposing any undue strain. In this instance the ultimate aim may not be to run continuously for 15 minutes, but for the participants to enjoy and benefit from the increased activity without being subjected to any stress. At the same time valuable leg strength is being maintained and even increased.

Try to jog on surfaces that give a little, like firm grass or a composite rubber surfaced running track, so reducing any jarring, strain and stress on joints. Jogging is good for stamina and helping control body weight, but it is not good for suppleness or upper body strength. When you are jogging over a distance there can be merit in stopping at a convenient point to walk a few yards and do a few stretching and loosening-up exercises, followed by a few gentle strides before continuing. There could also be merit in doing some upper body strengthening exercises on completion of your jogging session, to conclude with gentle mobility exercises in the warm-down.

If for some reason, perhaps due to work commitments or illness, you are not able to train for several days, it is advisable to recommence training at a less stressful stage of exercise than you were at when you left off. Beware of any continuous heavy or ponderous jogging action, for it can lead to joint strain and lower back pain. Your own instinct about how you feel should serve as a guide as to when to jog and walk. Regular exercise should be part of your long-range health programme and walking/jogging can make a valuable contribution to this aim.

## INTERVAL RUNNING

Interval running is a very effective form of training and suitable for the serious competitive athlete and sportsman. It involves bursts of maximum or near-maximum effort, alternating with short rest periods, such as running a specific distance (perhaps 50–1,000 yards) in a given time, or at a set effort, with short recovery periods between. As the bouts of intense physical activity are interspersed with short rest periods, the total work load achieved is much higher than would be possible in one continuous effort. This form of training will develop tolerance to oxygen debt and improve muscular endurance, strength and speed. When aimed at developing the capability to sustain effort it becomes a very serious form of endurance training, as recovery is not fully completed between each interval.

The principle used in interval training is that of 'overload'. Progression is normally achieved through extending the period of effort by increasing the number of intervals (repetitions) in a session; or the length of the resting period can be reduced, rather than raising the pace.

A simple example would be the endurance training, also related to speed, that is required by a rugby wing three-quarter who must have both pace and stamina for continuously sprinting in attack and covering in defence. His training schedule could include running three sets (see page 116) of three repetitions of 60-yard sprints at 90 per cent effort, broken halfway to perform two burpees (see page 218) to stimulate sudden stops and starts for tackles. Then, after walking back to the start point, he would repeat the sprint, but with a rest interval between each set. Gradually, after further training sessions and dependent on the player's fitness, the sprints could be increased to four or five per set, or the number of sets increased. The total repetitions possible will depend on a player's tolerance of this type of repetitive exercise and the degree of fitness he wishes to achieve. It is important that progressions are gradual to avoid injury to tendons and muscles. However, on a personal note, when training for rugby I found that with carefully graduated progressions I could eventually complete a total of twenty-six 60-yard sprints. This degree of endurance speed helped greatly when involved in chains of high-speed play and also in retaining skills when under stress, such as screw-kicking to touch or catching high balls.

Shortening the rest interval will also improve endurance. An example is where a club athlete is following a programme of running 4 x 400 metres at 80–90 per cent of maximum pace, perhaps with a rest interval of five minutes between each run. As he/she progresses, so the length of the rest interval would be reduced.

Different lengths of running intervals can result in different requirements and training effects. Short running intervals, as in sprinting, can be accomplished almost totally anaerobically. Long running intervals of four minutes and more have a high aerobic requirement and consequently a well-defined cardio-respiratory effect. Slope/hill running over inclines and descents at a fairly constant pace, perhaps for two to four minutes, combines the requirement for considerable anaerobic and cardio-respiratory efficiency with development of leg strength.

## Interval Training for Other Sports

Though interval running is much used by the serious competitive athlete, the principles can be adapted for use at any level. Meanwhile, the same principles that apply to interval running, involving bursts of maximum of near-maximum effort alternating with short rest periods, can also be applied to other sports such as swimming, rowing, canoeing and cycling.

### FARTLEK RUNNING

Fartlek running is a less formal type of interval training. The title is Scandinavian, derived from the Swedish words *fart* (speed) and *lek* (play). It involves a fairly lengthy training session of about 30 minutes, preferably through pleasant country such as forests, hills, fields, sand dunes or parks, carried out with many variations of pace. Fartlek running can either take the form of a programme aiming to create overload situations with built-in recovery phases, or can serve as a purposeful break from the monotony which is at times experienced with rigorous training. There might be pre-planned timed phases of jogging, fast-pace running, brisk walking, 50-yard sprint repetitions, striding and acceleration phases.

For even more relaxed training and, according to your mood, you could sprint up some slopes; walk a little; then jog to some distant landmark; stride down a slight incline; walk a little more; then sprint four 50-yard stretches with a jog between; stop in a glade and do some press-ups and sit-ups; and so on . . .

The concept of fartlek-type training is not reserved for the competitive athlete or the younger person, since it can be adapted for use by most ages and at various stages of fitness.

Some people may, according to their fitness, wish to walk at a modest pace for five minutes; then at a brisk pace for two minutes; stop to do a few gently rhythmic stretching exercises; trot for 50 or so paces; rest; then try a few angled press-ups, pressing up from the support of a felled tree or park bench; walk a little more; then, when you are ready, stride out for 20 paces; and so on . . .

## CYCLING

Cycling is an inexpensive way of getting around and seeing the countryside, places and people. As an exercise it is excellent for producing stamina and leg strength. Cycling also helps control body weight, though it does not make for flexibility. It can be enjoyed by all ages and, being weight-supporting, is a suitable activity for those overweight, though steep hills are best avoided. The bicycle is an amazing invention as it is the most effective known way of harnessing human muscle power. But because of this efficiency in terms of the energy used to cover a distance, it is necessary to cycle four miles to experience the training effect of running one mile. You therefore need to cycle some distance at a suitable constant speed to improve overall fitness; slow rides to work and back over short distances have but limited benefit.

### EQUIPMENT

There are now many types and models of cycle on the market, such as the high-handlebar single- or three-speed general purpose/shopping designs; five-speed sports roadsters; small-wheel folding models also with one or three speeds; mountain bikes suitable for very rugged terrain with up to 21 gears; and lightweight drop-handlebar touring and racing designs incorporating narrow tyres and a variety of gearing options.

However, when it comes to endurance training you can start on any bike that suits you. If you only possess a single-speed model, don't worry. It can serve as an excellent fitness training machine. You don't need to have a super expensive cycle to enjoy cycling or to cover a distance. Nurse Dervla Murphy rode a single-geared army bicycle from Ireland to India in the 1960s. It is on record that way back in 1880, H. Blackwell and C.A. Harman rode the length of Great Britain from Land's End to John o' Groats. They used penny-farthings!

If you are an older beginner then a general purpose bicycle could be what you want. The sports roadster and touring design are also options.

## Buying a Cycle

When buying a new cycle, find a bicycle shop that sells the type you want and allows a test ride. To determine the correct frame size, first of all straddle a sports roadster with your feet flat on the ground. If the size is correct the horizontal cross frame member should be about one inch below your crotch. When seated comfortably, the saddle should be adjusted so that when you push down on the pedals with the ball of the foot to the lowest point, your knee should be slightly bent. The handlebars need to be set at the right height for comfort and brakes and gear controls conveniently positioned.

## Clothing

For recreational cycling all you need is a pair of well-fitting shoes with a good firm rubber sole, worn with socks and slacks or shorts, plus a comfortable top. In the interest of safety, clothing should be colourful and reflective so that you can be seen by other road users. In cold weather clothing may need to be layered. In wet conditions a lightweight waterproof cape or anorak could be worn, with protective trousers. A cycling helmet is recommended, to give protection from serious injury in a collision or fall.

## Accessories

Accessories that need to be considered are a bell or horn to warn pedestrians, so safeguarding them and you, and goggles or wraparound sunglasses to keep flies and dust out of your eyes. A mileage indicator is a very useful addition and will help record an accurate log of your cycling trips. If you are going to cycle in built-up areas a rear-view mirror will enable you to see behind without the distraction of turning your head.

### BASIC CYCLING TECHNIQUE

A traffic-free park, playground or disused car park are ideal places to learn to ride a cycle and improve your technique.

First of all sit on the bike, your right foot on the right pedal that is raised forward, the left foot supporting on the ground. Set the bike in low gear. From the start always make the habit of looking behind you to check that the road is clear before you set off. Now push off with the left foot and begin to pedal. Effective and economical pedalling is dependent on the rider adopting a good riding position. With a flat-handlebar cycle sit with most of your body weight on the seat, but do not sit bolt upright. With a drop-handlebar cycle the rider needs to lean forward so that about half the body weight rests on the handlebars with the arms slightly bent.

As you pedal, exert pressure on the pedals with the ball of the foot, ensuring that the powerful lever action of the leg and foot is fully utilised. Avoid using the instep or the toes when pedalling, as less power is applied to the pedal in that case. As speed increases, change into a higher gear then, after a short distance, use the brakes gently to slow to a stop and start off again.

Once confidence is built up practise steering, perhaps between two parallel chalk lines marked on the ground about six inches apart. As you become more skilled, reduce the gap to four then two inches apart. Progress to practising cornering, gently at first, then leaning into the turn with the inside pedal raised to stop it hitting the ground. Safety procedures and a sound knowledge of the Highway Code (for hand signals, braking distances etc.) are of paramount importance to all

Figure 18: Basic Bicycle Designs

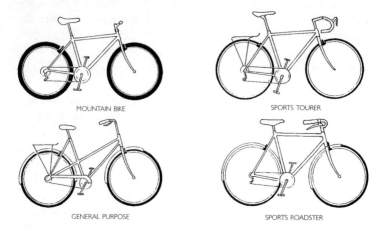

MOUNTAIN BIKE

SPORTS TOURER

GENERAL PURPOSE

SPORTS ROADSTER

cyclists. In many areas children can take cycling proficiency tests run by the road safety department of the local council.

## Pedal Cadence (Pedal Rate)

A smooth pedalling action at a constant suitable cadence makes for economy of effort and is of particular importance when pedalling a distance. Beginners may find that a pedal rate of about 60–70 revolutions per minute suits them, particularly if they are riding a general purpose or sports roadster. With practice, the fit younger cyclist riding a suitable lightweight design, should feel comfortable fanning the pedals at about 80–90 rpm. Whatever pedal rate is selected, the pace must allow you to be able to carry out a conversation with a companion, real or imaginary. When covering undulating ground, changing gear frequently makes for constant cadence, efficiency and reduced wear and tear on knees and muscles (and also on the cycle's chain and gears).

A simple way to check your cadence is to select a very quiet road, then with the use of a stopwatch or sweep-second hand, count the revolutions made in ten seconds and multiply by six. If your pedal rate is high, toe clips and straps will help take your legs through the full range of movement. These keep your foot in the correct position over the pedal, so increasing pedal power and making it easier to cycle uphill.

PROGRESSIVE TRAINING

There is a general tendency for fitness standards to be wrongly associated with vigorous competitive sport and the super-fit, rather than the lives of ordinary people. Such extreme standards can also be applied to cycling. The programmes that follow aim to give guidance to the beginner and the would-be cyclist of more modest ability. Progressions in a cycling programme can be achieved by gradually increasing the workload in a number of ways. Assuming that you have taken up cycling as an enjoyable recreational activity, but with an aim of improving your basic standard of fitness, here are some simple ways of achieving this aim. They follow the principle of overload by increasing the work rate, work duration and degree of resistance, and decreasing the recovery period. Whatever standard of cycling you are at, these principles can be adapted to help you progress.

PROGRESSIVE TWO-MILE CYCLING PROGRAMME This programme can be undertaken when a beginner is well used to his cycle and is capable of cycling for an hour or so. The programme aims to raise personal performance gradually by increasing work rate in preparation for longer periods of exercise that would have a definite aerobic effect. First of all, time yourself over a two-mile distance at a comfortable pace. This is your trial time (figure 19). The five examples give a wide range of cycling speed over the distance. Assuming, for the purpose of the exercise, that one of the five categories of cycling ability recorded fits your standard, aim to bring down your time over the two miles to the target time given for stage one through cycling every other day. Having achieved that target time, cycle a further two or three times at that speed to consolidate your improvement before aiming for the target time for stage two. Having achieved that target time, repeat the process through the remaining stages. Some people who are very fit, perhaps being also involved in weight training to develop leg power, may find the progressions insufficiently demanding. They would require greater time reductions at each stage – for example, by 20, 30 or more seconds instead of 15 seconds – but in all instances you should only progress to the next stage when you feel ready to do so.

As more target times are achieved, the effort required will become harder. The number of repetitions necessary may need to be increased before the next stage is reached; conversely, adjustments might require to be made to the programme to introduce gentler progressions. If at any time you cannot talk or whistle, slow down, for you are doing too much. As many individual time trials will not fit exactly into the five categories shown, compile your individual programme by following the pattern of progress outlined in figure 19, building in time reductions that suit. To estimate miles per hour, divide the time taken into 120 minutes.

Remember, we are aiming gradually to raise personal performance in preparation for longer periods of aerobic cycling. Adhere to the maxim 'train don't strain'. Steady practice through the two-mile programme should further test your cycling fitness and capability for future sustained cycling exercise.

Figure 19: Progressive Two-Mile Cycling Programme

| CATEGORY OF CYCLING ABILITY | I | II | III | IV | V |
|---|---|---|---|---|---|
| TWO-MILE TRIAL TIME (MINS AND SECS) | 16.00 | 14.00 | 10.30 | 9.00 | 8.00 |
| TARGET TIMES (MINS AND SECS) | | | | | |
| Stage 1 | 15.45 | 13.45 | 10.15 | 8.45 | 7.45 |
| Stage 2 | 15.30 | 13.30 | 10.00 | 8.30 | 7.30 |
| Stage 3 | 15.15 | 13.15 | 9.45 | 8.15 | 7.15 |
| Stage 4 | 15.00 | 13.00 | 9.30 | 8.00 | 7.00 |
| Stage 5 | 14.45 | 12.45 | 9.15 | 7.45 | 6.45 |
| APPROXIMATE MPH FOR STAGE 5 | 8 | 9½ | 13 | 16 | 18½ |

PACE/TIME/DISTANCE PROGRAMME The aim of this programme is to improve endurance capability by increasing the work rate and reducing recovery periods in each stage of training. You should exercise every other day and progress to the next stage only when you are ready.

Stage
1. Cycle at moderate pace for 30 minutes. Measure and record the distance covered.
2. Cycle for 12 minutes at moderate pace, then about six minutes at a brisk pace, to conclude with 12 minutes at moderate pace.
3. Cycle for ten minutes at moderate pace, then five minutes at brisk pace, then ten more minutes at moderate pace, ending with another five minutes at brisk pace.
4. Cycle for five minutes at moderate pace, then five minutes at brisk pace, then continue to alternate the same pace variation over the 30-minute session.
5. Cycle for five minutes at moderate pace, then ten minutes at brisk pace and continue the sequence over the exercise session.
6. Cycle for about 12 minutes at brisk pace, then about six minutes at a moderate pace, to conclude with 12 minutes at brisk pace.
7. Cycle for 30 minutes at brisk pace, then measure and record the distance covered.

Further progressions can be made by extending the cycling time and applying the same principles of increasing the work rate and reducing the recovery periods.

INCLINE CYCLING Once you have become cycling fit by cycling on mainly flat terrain it may be time to change to more undulating roads and lanes. This will involve increased resistance training. Many inclines are not obvious to the car driver, but a long gradual ascent on a bicycle involves working against gravity and can make considerable demands on the cyclist. The result is an increased aerobic capacity. Your local area may provide some inclines or hills that can be used to increase your fitness, so be aware of the local topography.

The use of different gears at the appropriate point on ascents is important. As you approach an incline, change down one or more gears to maintain your pedalling rate. Modern multi-geared cycles allow the rider to climb quite steep slopes; but three- and five-speed gear models are still popular in many countries, though they can be harder to pedal on more severe inclines. However if the effort is too great at any time, particularly if you are a beginner or an older person, and whether it be in early stages of training or even later, get off the bike, walk or perhaps have a rest before you continue.

Whatever form of gearing you have on your bike, when covering a familiar training route it is useful to identify distinctive features on the ascent that can serve as gear change points. As leg strength and general fitness improves while practice over the route is repeated, it will eventually be possible to change the points at which you change gear higher up the hill, giving proof of your increased fitness.

The example in figure 20 incorporates, for simplicity, the use of a three-geared cycle and shows an incline with features alongside a lane – a country inn and two trees. The actual gear change points for the three-geared bike during the ascent are also shown. Initially the gear change points are well down the slope and made at the position of the features (20A). At this stage of fitness the cyclist eventually has to dismount and walk up the most severe part of the ascent. With further cycling practice and a higher standard of fitness, it is possible to change gear higher up the slope, midway between the features, though the cyclist still has to dismount at the steepest part (20B). Eventually, after attaining greater cycling fitness, it is possible to use the two trees as gear change points for third to second and second to first gear respectively, which results in the slope being cleared without dismounting (20C). In due course it may be possible to clear the slope in second or even third gear. However, never hesitate to drop down a gear at any time to avoid strain on joints and tendons.

Where there is a descent ahead, test the brakes before making a run down the slope. Change up the gears as you

Figure 20: Incline Cycling (using limited gearing)

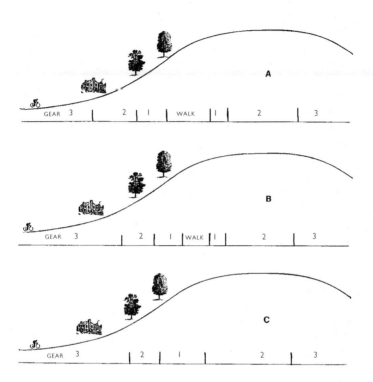

accelerate, then freewheel to rest the legs, braking as necessary from time to time to keep the speed under control. When close to the bottom of the descent, resume pedalling to maintain your speed.

When riding steep inclines it may be necessary to seek extra power. One way is to grip the handlebars firmly, rise out of the saddle to stand on the pedals and swing the cycle from side to side beneath you, using your body weight to reinforce the muscular effort applied. This is known as 'honking'. Another technique used by fit cyclists to surmount short steep hills is known as 'ankling'. Here additional power from the ankle is employed for much of the rotational pedal movement. The ankle is dorsi-flexed (foot pointed up) on the commencement of the pedals

93

descent, then planter-flexed (foot pressed to point down) to bring extra pressure on the pedal through a considerable part of its circular movement.

Cycling is an inexpensive way of touring, enabling you to see, hear and enjoy the countryside at your own pace. A tour for near-beginners should be planned through an area of interest over suitable cycling terrain and describe a circle. Start in the middle of the circle, aiming to cover about 20 to 30 miles a day. This is a manageable distance for a reasonably fit cyclist and allows time for sightseeing and rests. Such a plan ensures that in the event of an emergency, the starting point will never be too far away.

To sum up, cycling is a convenient way of getting around and enjoying the outdoors. An environment-friendly means of transport, it presents no parking problems and enables the rider to explore places that cars cannot reach. Regular cycling helps to prolong life. It provides little stress on joints and therefore can be enjoyed by a wide range of body types. It has many fitness benefits, the most important of which is the development of aerobic fitness. Cycling is a very pleasurable activity suitable for all the family.


## SWIMMING

Swimming is an excellent form of exercise. It improves aerobic fitness, promotes strength by exercising the major muscles of the upper and lower body and makes for flexibility. Swimming is a non-stressful, low injury-risk activity as the body is supported by the water and there is neither jarring nor pounding during exercise. It is therefore an ideal form of exercise to pursue if you are overweight, or undergoing a period of recovery from injury, particularly when suffering from injury to the back or legs (though those with a neck injury should avoid the breaststroke). The support that the water gives also enables the swimmer to concentrate and put all his effort into the exercise, instead of having to divert some energy in adopting the upright posture as is required in games, walking or running.

The rate of energy utilisation in recreational swimming is comparatively low, being just half that of jogging. Therefore swimming as a recreation will have very little effect on weight reduction. The aerobic training effect will depend on how long the training sessions last, their intensity and the frequency with which they are repeated. Nevertheless, swimming carried out for long periods, even just at a slow plodding pace, can have aerobic benefits. It is not necessary to be a master of swimming strokes to ensure improvement in aerobic capacity. An experienced breaststroke swimmer can continue almost indefinitely, barely using more energy than in walking but resulting in an improvement in endurance. Switching to other strokes will bring in different muscles and make for added flexibility. This variation also helps to reduce boredom when swimming some distance.

Perhaps the main problem when considering swimming as a form of aerobic exercise is that many people do not have the ability to swim sufficiently well to keep going and to maintain a heart rate that will have a training effect. It is also an area of exercise where personal ability varies greatly. Some are able to streak up and down the pool with comparatively little effort, while others have to work very hard, yet cannot match the former's pace and take double the time to cover the same distance. What matters is the overall amount of energy used: the training effect may be the same for both categories of swimmers despite the difference in performance.

## HOW TO START

Swimming is an activity that can, like walking and cycling, be enjoyed well into old age. It is never too late to learn to swim or to improve your swimming ability. Swimming requires confidence, correct breathing, rhythm and regular practice. If possible swim every other day; once you can swim four or five lengths it will not be long before you can swim continuously.

Basic training programmes can take various forms. The most simple would be to set yourself a goal, perhaps to aim to swim continuously for ten or 15 minutes without stopping. Begin slowly and gently, paying attention to good form and correct breathing, swimming three or four times a week. Perhaps you can only swim a couple of lengths to start with. Have a rest, then see if you can swim further. Gradually increase the number of lengths that you can swim and also reduce the length of rest periods. Once you have reached your initial goal of swimming constantly for ten or 15 minutes, reset your goal to swim for an extra five or more minutes.

SWIMMING ABILITY TEST A more challenging form of progressive programme covers 20 minutes. If you can, start at level two.

Level 1 Begin slowly and gently and swim three to four times a week. According to the progress made add one minute or more a week (or when you are ready) to the time you swim until you can swim for 20 minutes. Now go to level 2.

Level 2 First of all record how many lengths you swam in 20 minutes. Now swim a little more vigorously, gradually increasing the number of lengths you can cover in the same time. Initially you may see a fair improvement, but as you continue progress will become more difficult. When you cannot record any further improvement over three consecutive session move on to level 3.

Level 3 Further progressions can take various forms. Examples are as follows:
a. Swim for a progressively longer period of time by adding one or two minutes at the end of each week or every two weeks.
b. Add an extra length of the pool each week.
c. Vary your strokes, perhaps by alternating three lengths breaststroke, two backstroke and one crawl.

d.Vary the speed of your training by swimming a fast
length followed by a slow recovery length and then
repeat the sequence.

PROGRESSIVE TRAINING FOR A DISTANCE SWIM **Figure 21 gives an example**
of a simple personal 12-week/stage action plan for a modest
ability recreational swimmer to attain the goal of swimming
800 yards in under 19 minutes. It is based on gradually
increasing the distance swum per week/stage against a set
time, but at a constant pace. Move to the next progression at
the end of each week, or when you are ready. The distance is
increased by 50 yards per week/stage over the first eight
weeks/stages; then, as the swimmer has built up endurance
and improved his technique, increased to 100 yards per
week/stage over the remaining four weeks/stages. If the 100-
yard increase per week/stage included in the last four weeks
is too demanding, the progressions for this phase could be
adjusted accordingly and substituted by 50-yard stages.
According to your ability and personal aim, such a plan can
easily be adapted to meet your individual requirements of
time and distance. See figure 7 to record your progress.

Figure 21: Progressive Swimming Training Plan

| WEEK/STAGE | DISTANCE (YARDS) | DURATION (MINUTES/SECONDS) |
|:---:|:---:|:---:|
| 1 | 50 | 1.10 |
| 2 | 100 | 2.20 |
| 3 | 150 | 3.30 |
| 4 | 200 | 4.40 |
| 5 | 250 | 5.50 |
| 6 | 300 | 7.00 |
| 7 | 350 | 8.10 |
| 8 | 400 | 9.20 |
| 9 | 500 | 11.40 |
| 10 | 600 | 14.00 |
| 11 | 700 | 16.20 |
| 12 | 800 | 18.40 |

Some people are not able to cope with such strokes as the front crawl and butterfly. They may feel these strokes are too advanced. Perhaps they dislike putting their face into the water and having to use the breathing techniques required. Those prone to asthma can experience difficulties in this area. The breaststroke carried out with the face out of the water is a stroke that avoids these problems.

There are two more strokes – one performed on the back, the other on the side – that are no longer fashionable or feasible in competitive swimming but could be employed by the recreational swimmer who prefers to keep mouth and eyes clear of the water. They are also worth learning for adaptation to lifesaving techniques. Both require comparatively little energy, can be performed over a distance and are not difficult to learn. Each is described below with a variation.

## Backstroke

ENGLISH BACKSTROKE (figure 22) The swimmer lies horizontally on his back with his face clear of the water (A). The sequence of the arm and leg actions can be carried out as follows:

a. The arms are raised together high over the water and placed, hands almost touching, palms facing outwards, in the water above the head (B). At the same time the legs are drawn up so that the knees form an approximate right angle with the feet together (C). Breathe in during the movement.
b. Propulsion is effected by the arms describing a wide sculling action, the palms gaining purchase on the water as they are swept down to the thighs. The leg kick, which resembles an inverted breaststroke, is made simultaneously (D). The leg action describes an arc, the inside of the legs and feet pushing against the water as the legs are squeezed together to give propulsion. Breathe out during the movement.
c. The simultaneous arm sweep and leg kick ends in the

Figure 22: Easy Strokes for Recreational Swimming – English Backstroke

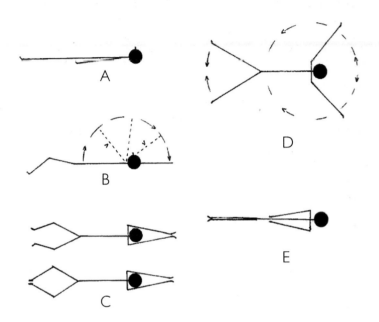

streamline body position to effect a glide (E) before the movement is repeated.

ELEMENTARY BACKSTROKE This is a modern version of the English backstroke in which the arm recovery is made under the water. As with the English backstroke, the swimmer lies horizontally on his back with his face clear of the water. The sequence of the arm and leg action is as follows:

a. The hands are moved up underneath the water from the side of the thighs to the chest, then fully extended sideways in line with the shoulders. At the same time the legs are drawn up and the knees bent by dropping the lower leg. The heels are about hip width apart. Breathe in during this simultaneous movement.

b. Propulsion from the arms is gained by sweeping the arms in a wide sculling action down to the thighs with the palms extended to catch the water. The simultaneous leg kick is similar to that of an inverted breaststroke. Breathe out as the propulsion action takes place.

c. The simultaneous arm sweep and leg kick ends in the streamline body position to make the glide before repeating the sequence.

### Sidestrokes

The second swimming stroke that poses little breathing difficulty is the sidestroke. Two types are described, the traditional sidestroke and the conventional sidestroke. The traditional sidestroke was popular many years ago, before the introduction of the front crawl as we know it by Johnny Weismuller, the original Tarzan of the films and one-time Olympic swimming champion. It was used for both racing and long-distance swimming and was one of the strokes that carried the redoubtable Captain Matthew Webb on many of his epic swimming ventures. None was greater than that of the first-ever crossing of the English Channel from Dover to Calais in August 1875. Webb swam 38 miles against the currents to make the 21-mile crossing in 21 hours and 45 minutes.

The traditional conventional sidestrokes may assist the less capable swimmer to swim for longer and further and, in so doing, increase his/her aerobic fitness. The economy of effort of the traditional sidestroke was proven to me on a military exercise when I used to swim the length of the Eider See in Germany, which is several miles long.

TRADITIONAL SIDESTROKE (figure 23) The swimmer lies on one side in the water, described here as the right side, with the head resting on the water, and eyes, nose and mouth clear of the surface. The sequence of the arm and leg actions are as follows:

Figure 23: Easy Strokes for Recreational Swimming – Traditional Sidestroke

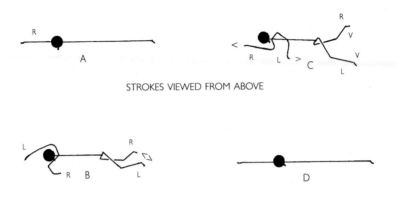

STROKES VIEWED FROM ABOVE

a. The right arm is extended fully forward with fingers pointed (A). Initial arm propulsion is made by the right hand catching the water as the hand is drawn back to the chest. As it does so the left arm is advanced over the water, fingers cupped to enter the surface beyond the head (B).

b. The leg action comprises the simultaneous parting of the legs with the knees bent as the left arm is advanced, the upper leg moving forward, the lower leg backward (B). Leg propulsion results from the legs being swept together and straightened in a powerful scissor kick as the left arm makes its stroke, resembling the action of the front crawl, with the hand being recovered alongside the body as the right arm is extended forward (C). The streamlined position now assumed, with the right arm extended, is retained for the glide (D). The movements are repeated.

c. Breathing in takes place as the right arm is extended forward, the head turning slightly to look back, the bow wave formed leaving the mouth clear to allow unimpeded breathing (D). Breathing out takes place when the body turns slightly as the left arm is advanced to strike and enter the water.

CONVENTIONAL SIDESTROKE This is a simpler and more common

stroke than the traditional sidestroke. It starts in the same way with the swimmer lying on his side in the water, here also described as the right side, head resting on the surface, eyes, nose and mouth clear of the water. The sequence of arm and leg movements are then as follows:

a. The right arm is extended fully forward with fingers pointed. Initial propulsion is effected by the right hand being drawn downwards and sideways to the chest as the left arm is moved forward under the water, elbow bent to a position where the hand is below the head. Continuing the simultaneous movement, the left hand pushes down and back to the thigh to effect further arm propulsion while the right arm recovers to the extended position out in front.

b. The leg action comprises the simultaneous parting of the legs with the knees bent, the upper leg moving forward and the lower backward, and occurs as the right hand is drawn back. Leg propulsion results from the legs being swept together and straightened in a powerful scissor kick as the left arm makes its stroke and the right arm is extended forward. The streamlined position is now assumed with the right arm extended and the left arm, held at the side, retained for the glide.

c. Breathing in takes place as the propulsive sweep of the right arm is made which tends to lift the shoulders and head. Breathing out takes place as the glide commences.

In summary, swimming is one of the cheapest forms of exercise. It can be performed alone but also has social advantages. It is not an activity that must be reluctantly given up with the onset of the years and it can be enjoyed quietly, without undue strain or fatigue. Swimming is an activity that can benefit people with physical disabilities. In the rehabilitation of the injured it can play an important part in treating those suffering from muscular disorders. Great pleasure can also be derived from swimming by the blind, deaf and dumb as well as people with learning difficulties. It is therefore an activity that has competitive, recreational, therapeutic and aerobic benefits. With very wide appeal, it is suitable for all the family.

## CIRCUIT TRAINING

Circuit training is a popular and proven method of fitness training that is suitable not only for team or class training, but also for individual practice. It is an effective means of developing endurance, but has the added advantage that strength, speed, skill and suppleness can be improved through the inclusion of exercises which have these specific aims.

Circuit training comprises a series of vigorous exercises performed in a particular sequence in order to involve the different parts of the body. It uses apparatus or body resistance and is planned in a circular arrangement that permits progressions from one exercise station to another until all the stations have been visited. Different muscle groups are therefore used each time. This allows other groups to recover and the high intensity work load to be maintained. The result is a beneficial effect on the heart and lungs.

Circuits normally involve the use of benches, medicine balls, mats, perhaps pull-up bars or gymnasium beams, but they can be devised using little or no equipment. Therefore circuit training is suitable for consideration in a home exercise programme (see page 191).

INITIAL TESTING

An exercise circuit can involve some six to twelve different exercises. First of all, practise each exercise to ensure correct technique. The individual is then tested on each exercise to establish his/her personal training level. This is done by recording the total number of repetitions possible that can be performed in one minute on each exercise. The repetitions need not be performed continuously throughout the minute: for example, an individual may do 20 sit-ups, then rest for several seconds before completing six or more within the minute, so carrying out a total of 26 sit-ups. Adequate rest periods are allowed between exercises.

## Training Level

The training level for working around the circuit continuously is half the maximum number of repetitions recorded for each exercise, i.e. the individual who managed 26 sit-ups would be required to perform 13 sit-ups.

## A Circuit

On a given signal, individuals begin to work around the circuit, operating at their own individual training levels by performing half their maximum repetitions for each respective exercise. Three to five laps are accomplished, each lap being timed with one or more minutes' rest between circuits (or more, according to the individual's fitness). Each training session lasts for 20–30 minutes. The programme should be undertaken three times a week.

Progression is achieved by reducing the time taken to complete each lap and by increasing the number of laps. A good stimulus is to aim for a one-quarter reduction in lap time. After a set number of exercise sessions, individuals can be retested to check the maximum repetitions per minute they can now perform at each exercise station. Their training level is then adjusted. Figure 24 shows an eight-station circuit-training programme. Figure 25 is a prepared circuit-training record card relating to that programme. A variation in progression that can be more suited to the home exerciser is given under Home Circuit Training on page 193.

Figure 24: Eight-Station Circuit-Training Programme

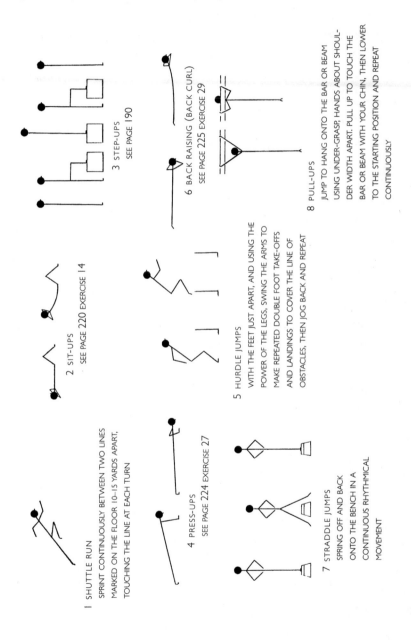

3 STEP-UPS
SEE PAGE 190

6 BACK RAISING (BACK CURL)
SEE PAGE 225 EXERCISE 29

8 PULL-UPS
JUMP TO HANG ONTO THE BAR OR BEAM
USING UNDER-GRASP, HANDS ABOUT SHOUL-
DER WIDTH APART. PULL UP TO TOUCH THE
BAR OR BEAM WITH YOUR CHIN, THEN LOWER
TO THE STARTING POSITION AND REPEAT
CONTINUOUSLY

2 SIT-UPS
SEE PAGE 220 EXERCISE 14

5 HURDLE JUMPS
WITH THE FEET JUST APART, AND USING THE
POWER OF THE LEGS, SWING THE ARMS TO
MAKE REPEATED DOUBLE FOOT TAKE-OFFS
AND LANDINGS TO COVER THE LINE OF
OBSTACLES, THEN JOG BACK AND REPEAT

1 SHUTTLE RUN
SPRINT CONTINUOUSLY BETWEEN TWO LINES
MARKED ON THE FLOOR 10–15 YARDS APART,
TOUCHING THE LINE AT EACH TURN

4 PRESS-UPS
SEE PAGE 224 EXERCISE 27

7 STRADDLE JUMPS
SPRING OFF AND BACK
ONTO THE BENCH IN A
CONTINUOUS RHYTHMICAL
MOVEMENT

Figure 25: Circuit-Training Record Card (Eight Stations)

| | | WEEKLY TRAINING LEVEL | | | | | |
|---|---|---|---|---|---|---|---|
| EXERCISE | PURPOSE | 1 | 2 | 3 | 4 | 5 | 6 |
| Shuttle run | For speed, agility and stamina | | | | | | |
| Sit-ups | For abdominal strength | | | | | | |
| Step-ups | For leg strength and endurance | | | | | | |
| Press-ups | For arm and shoulder strength | | | | | | |
| Hurdle jumps | For leg power | | | | | | |
| Back raising | For back strength | | | | | | |
| Straddle jumps | For leg power and stamina | | | | | | |
| Pull-ups | For arm and shoulder strength | | | | | | |

## TRIM TRAILS

In their quest for fitness many people take to health clubs to gain the benefits of personal instruction; or they are attracted by the lycra image and state-of-the-art equipment, plus the social side with the exclusive if expensive status that some clubs afford. Other people prefer a more individual, though equally dedicated, approach to exercise and seek to avoid formal instruction in what might be crowded gymnasiums.

There is no doubt that you do not need weights or expensive training machines to perform an effective work-out. Right at hand can be the cheapest and most available health club in the world. It is called the 'Great Outdoors'. It has enjoyable benefits. There is nothing to beat exercising in the fresh air, whether it be in sunshine, the cool of the evening or even in the rain. Exercising outdoors is exhilarating. It gives the complexion a healthy glow and the body an overall glorious feeling of well-being. The natural facilities of the outdoors can, with a little planning, provide highly effective exercise opportunities to meet all our training requirements, yet be available in a tranquil environment that gives relief from the hustle, pressures and anxieties of daily life.

Figure 26: Trim Trails – Suitable Exercises

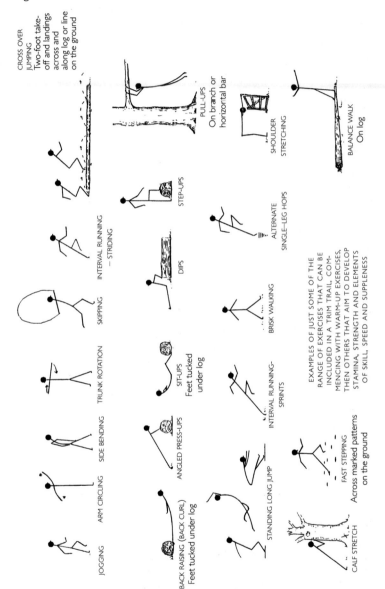

CROSS OVER JUMPING Two-foot take-off and landings across and along log or line on the ground

PULL-UPS On branch or horizontal bar

SHOULDER STRETCHING

BALANCE WALK On log

STEP-UPS

INTERVAL RUNNING – STRIDING

SKIPPING

DIPS

ALTERNATE SINGLE-LEG HOPS

TRUNK ROTATION

SIDE BENDING

SIT-UPS Feet tucked under log

BRISK WALKING

ARM CIRCLING

ANGLED PRESS-UPS

INTERVAL RUNNING-SPRINTS

JOGGING

BACK RAISING (BACK CURL) Feet tucked under log

STANDING LONG JUMP

FAST STEPPING Across marked patterns on the ground

CALF STRETCH

EXAMPLES OF JUST SOME OF THE RANGE OF EXERCISES THAT CAN BE INCLUDED IN A TRIM TRAIL, COMMENCING WITH WARM-UP EXERCISES, THEN OTHERS THAT AIM TO DEVELOP STAMINA, STRENGTH AND ELEMENTS OF SKILL, SPEED AND SUPPLENESS

Some local leisure authorities have laid out interesting, attractive trim trails in parks and recreational areas. These normally comprise a circular course with numerous exercise stops (stations) giving the opportunity to perform set exercises at these points – perhaps using logs, rustic benches, pull-up bars, balance logs or bars. The exercises are arranged in a particular sequence so as to involve the different muscle groups and, according to the type of exercises, the repetitions performed and resistance involved can have aerobic or strengthening effects or elements of both.

Some trim tracks are graded in difficulty so as to accommodate different fitness and ability levels. For example, after a warm-up of your choice, you might commence by jogging to the first station; then stop to carry out chair dips on a log; move on to sit-ups with feet held by a low bar or log; jog to a pull-up bar; and do step-ups on a rustic bench. Now stride and sprint alternately between the oak trees; then walk a while before balance-walking forwards and backwards on a low bar or log; and stride around the lake. Finally, warm down with gentle stretching exercises, some performed against a tree trunk or gate.

If you find, after enquiring at your local leisure department, that there are no trim trails in the area, have a thought as to how you can plan your own. Figure 26 gives examples of some of the exercises that could be included in a trim trail.

# SIX

# Exercising for Strength

The possession of an aesthetic physique has always been admired and much sought after by both males and females. The sculptures of ancient times exemplify good posture, balanced musculature and strength. Judged by the current popularity of health clubs and the desire to 'look good', interest in the area of body development has reached new levels, much focusing on body improvement through strength training. However, you do not need to join an expensive city gym in order to firm up muscles. An understanding of the types of equipment necessary, training methods, basic techniques and safety precautions will help decide how and where you can exercise for strength.

Today's scientific approach to strength training, based on progressive resistance, contributes greatly to the athletic feats and performances now being recorded. It also contributes to success in the fields of medical rehabilitation. But strength training has not been confined to modern times. Over the centuries strength played an important part in our ancestors' lives. For example, evidence of the personal strength of the 5,000 archers who fought at the Battle of Agincourt in 1415 was confirmed in the 1980s when perfectly preserved six-foot longbows were raised with the wreck of the Mary Rose galleon. When the bows, similar to those used at Agincourt, were tested it was found that each bow required the upper body and arm strength to pull 180 lb! Furthermore, each archer was capable of drawing and releasing 15 well-aimed arrows per minute, and firing continuously up to 330 yards.

Most of these men were freemen with smallholdings who lived off the land. Their work was manual and their physical development was furthered by mandatory weekly archery practice at the local 'butts'. Such practice commenced at an early age with low-powered bows and progressed by increasing the workload through the use of stronger bows to the formidable 'battle bow'. Few people of our time would be able to draw such a weapon!

In more recent times, but before the introduction of modern coal-cutting machinery, much of the coal-miners' work was manual and they often worked in narrow seams. Every hour of their long working shifts demanded strength, suppleness and endurance. In South Wales their remarkable fitness was often honed to perfection by two rugby training sessions a week and a game on Saturday. The miner was a most formidable rugby opponent. The power he possessed – demonstrated by his body strength, agility, steel-like sinews and vice-like grip, to which was added great determination – is well remembered by those who played in the Welsh Valleys or against Welsh clubs at the time. There are now few vocations that demand such a high degree of fitness.

How, then, can we develop strength? It has been defined as the muscular force that can be applied with a single maximum effort against a resistance. Training for increased strength depends upon building muscle bulk by repeated work against the resistance of heavy loads. All forms of training involve making muscles work. In aerobic exercise many muscles are worked at the same time and together, but with no particular group experiencing a heavy load. In this form of training it is possible to repeat movements many times, so improving the capacity to endure sustained continuous exercise of a moderate intensity. Such exercise develops the muscles' slow twitch fibres (see page 38). However, in strength training the aim is to involve a comparatively small number of muscles at a time, but to subject them to much heavier loads. The level of the load limits the number of repetitions possible. In this form of training muscle power is improved by developing fast twitch muscles fibres (see page 37).

Strength can be achieved by using our body weight, as in push-ups; or by the use of apparatus such as weights, springs, pulleys and hydraulics. Whatever system is used, for a muscle to become stronger it must be put in a state of overload. This is done by selecting resistance heavy enough to ensure that the muscle works sufficiently hard to a set capacity. At that stage the resistance is increased, ensuring the further development of strength, and the process is repeated. To gain the benefits of strength, training exercises should involve a resistance that limits the number of repetitive movements to no more than ten or twelve.

Whether you are looking for an improvement in muscle tone or to serious body building, equipment is available in many forms.

Weight-Training Equipment

There are two principal types of weight-training equipment: free weights, such as bar-bells and dumb-bells; and training machines (see pages 228ff.).

FREE WEIGHTS The bar-bell comprises a five- to seven-foot solid steel bar on which adjustable discs made of iron, often vinyl covered, are held in place by collars. They are intended for two-handed lifting or pushing actions. The dumb-bell is a shorter bar of eight to 14 inches and can take the same form as the bar-bell with adjustable discs and securing collars, or can be constructed in moulded form in vinyl at a set weight, being filled with aggregate. Dumb-bells are used mainly for single or simultaneous double-arm actions. Though the use of free weights initially requires instruction and practice in their use, they are ideal for the individual who enjoys this type of exercise, offering a great variety of movement with beneficial effects on muscle control, balance and co-ordination.

TRAINING MACHINES Weight-training machines, or multi-gyms, are now very popular and are to be found in most sports centres. They are usually large pieces of equipment. The exercises are carried out by pulling or pushing a handle or lever, or by controlling the movement of weights through a pulley. These are fully adjustable by moving a screw or peg, allowing you to increase or decrease weights and resistance to meet your own capabilities. Multi-gyms that incorporate a bench press are generally the most versatile; seated press-style multi-gyms are normally the most space efficient. The weight-training machine comprises a number of stations and the participant moves from station to station, exercising different muscle groups in a set order. Though they make for relatively safe operation and their use is normally quickly understood, they often allow only fairly limited types of movement through fixed arcs. Correspondingly, the degree of improved muscular control and co-ordination may be less than that experienced with the use of free weights. However, training machines are well suited for use by the individual or teams in developing strength as part of training for a specific sport.

VARIATIONS IN STRENGTH-TRAINING MACHINES AND EQUIPMENT The muscle power curve is the varying force that a muscle can exert at different muscle lengths. When free weights are used the muscle can be either underloaded in the middle range of a movement, or overloaded at the extremes of the movement.

This recognition of strength variation at different positions during a movement has brought about much research and influenced the design of modern weight-training equipment. 'Isokinetic' training machines are designed to ensure that the speed of exercise levers is constant and resistance is varied according to the strength of the muscle, so maintaining high tension throughout the range of the movement. Other strength-training machines involve working against hydraulic pistons and are based on the principle that the more vigorous the movements made, the greater the resistance encountered. Despite these comparatively recent developments, many authorities consider the use of free weights an excellent way of gaining strength. Other training machines and devices on the market range from chest expanders and rowing machines to the popular Bullworker isotonic and isometric exerciser.

## Training Systems

As stated in chapter 1 under Components of Fitness, strength can be demonstrated as static strength (involving isometric resistance), explosive strength and dynamic strength (involving isotonic muscle action). The object in strength training is to force the muscle involved to recruit as many muscle fibres as possible in a single contraction. If this is achieved and the maximum number of fibres brought into play, the muscle will adapt by increasing the thickness of the individual fibres. Various systems aim to achieve maximum fibre recruitment using different types of equipment and different forms of muscle contraction.

ISOTONIC EXERCISE SYSTEMS Free weights are a traditional method of increasing strength applied through concentric muscle work (where muscles shorten) and eccentric muscle work (where muscles lengthen), for example when lifting a weight and then lowering it back to the start position as with two-hand curls. A muscle working concentrically shortens and thickens with the origin and insertion of the muscle moving towards each other. When working eccentrically the origin

113

and insertion of the muscle move away from one another. The muscle becomes longer and thinner, paying out gradually to control the movement (see figure 27).

In isotonic training, repeated movements are made with a weight heavy enough to recruit a considerable number of fibres. As the muscle becomes fatigued, more muscle fibres are recruited.

ISOMETRIC EXERCISE SYSTEMS It is believed that isometric muscle contractions, where the muscle length does not change as the muscle is in contraction against an immovable resistance, ensures the maximum recruitment of fibres possible (pages 25 and 203). The origin and insertion of the muscle do not move and there is also no movement in the joint. For example, when holding a heavy bucket of water up high with two hands, the elbow joints are fixed and the elbow flexors, working statically, maintain the position. For maximum effect isometric contractions should be made at strongest effort and last for six seconds (page 204 gives essential initial progressions). Isometric systems can employ the use of springs, heavy weights and pushing or attempting to lift immovable objects. The limitations of isometric exercise is that they are static and develop strength in but one fixed position, though if increased strength is sought throughout a range of movement, exercises can be performed at angles within the range. Isometric exercises can limit flexibility and therefore need to be accompanied by mobility exercises. They have a limiting effect on the circulation and can, during exercise, increase blood pressure. Figure 46 (page 206) gives examples of this type of training.

## How to Start

Before you start exercising with weights, whether using free weights or multi-station units, you should seek the guidance of a qualified instructor – who is normally readily available at most sports centres – so as to make yourself thoroughly familiar with the techniques of weight training and the safety precautions necessary.

Figure27: Muscle Action

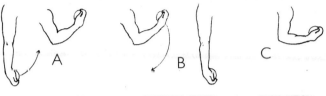

CONCENTRIC ACTION      ECCENTRIC ACTION      STATIC ACTION

ACTION OF THE BICEPS MUSCLE (FRONT OF UPPER ARM) WHEN A LIFTING A
WEIGHT AND WORKING CONCENTRICALLY; B WHEN LOWERING A WEIGHT
WORKING ECCENTRICALLY; AND C HOLDING THE WEIGHT WORKING STATICALLY.

SAFETY **Weight training can be dangerous unless sensible safety
procedures are observed. Note the following points:**

a. Before you start training make sure you have a good
warm-up to include flexibility exercises so that the
body is well prepared for the schedule to follow.

b. Seek expert advice if you are going to use unfamiliar
equipment, perform an unfamiliar exercise, or are in
any way unsure how to use the equipment.

c. Check all apparatus before and after use. Make sure that
collars are secure, bars are evenly balanced and that
equipment is safe and well maintained.

d. Make sure that there is adequate space, that the floor of
the training area is firm and non-slip and that your
footwear is suitable.

e. When starting an unfamiliar exercise, use light weights
initially so that you can concentrate on carrying out
the movement correctly, including correct breathing,
before adding greater weight.

f. Avoid exercises or body positions that may damage vulnerable parts of the body, e.g. lower back and knee joints.

g. When using heavy weights never train alone. Have a
stand-in at the end of each bar who understands the
exercise and his/her own safety role.

h. If pain is experienced in the working muscles or joints,
*stop exercising.*

All weight training is based on repetitions, sets and resistance amplified as follows:

REPETITIONS A repetition (rep) is a single execution of an exercise, normally given as the number of times that an exercise is carried out continuously, for instance 15 reps.

SETS A set is a group of continuous repetitions of an exercise. Three sets of 12 repetitions would be recorded as 3 x 12.

RESISTANCE Resistance is the load that the muscle or muscle group has to move. If in the form of weight, it is normally indicated in kilograms.

Your initial aim should be to develop general strength. If in due course you are to specialise in one particular sport or game, your training with weights should eventually relate to that activity. For example, a javelin thrower would aim to develop explosive arm and shoulder power plus general all-round body strength; a rugby front-row forward would wish to develop upper body strength in addition to general body strength. Once the muscle groups that will be involved in your sport are identified, specific exercises can be planned (see page 120, Weight-Training Exercises for Sport).

A Basic Weight-Training Programme

Because there are so many variations in the physical build of individuals, plus differences in age and ability, it is impossible to be precise as to the actual weight of dumb-bells or bar-bells to be used. This is best decided by the instructor. However, a weight selected should permit the movement to be learnt but also exercise the participant. According to age and fitness, it can be as low as 5 lb (2.2 kg) or less, perhaps also being suitable for remedial patients; or 15 lb (7 kg) to 30 lb (14 kg) or much more. The beginner should note that the weight selected for initial training may seem quite light, but the workload may demand sets of 15 repetitions or more and a fair degree of effort. A weight training programme should have a balanced sequence of exercises that will exercise muscle groups in rotation – such as legs, chest, back, shoulders, arms and abdominals. Practise using a light load that you can handle with ease and concentrate on technique. Now increase to a modest load to commence initial training that will permit, say, 15 reps, although these may vary per exercise and depend on the strength of the muscles being used. Each exercise should be performed in a well-controlled movement with a steady rhythm. With a few exceptions, it is advisable to inhale as you lift the weight and to exhale as it is lowered. Avoid holding your breath, as this compresses the chest and can produce high intrathoracic pressure which prevents the venous return of blood to the heart and may result in dizziness or feeling faint. Also check that each exercise is being performed with the body in the correct balanced position.

PROGRESSION After a suitable number of training sessions the resistance/weights should be increased to a load that will allow but ten to 12 reps. Ideally strength training should take place every other day, perhaps with six exercises in each programme. Progress can be made as follows:

a. Once the first series of the six exercises has been completed, a short rest of about two minutes is taken and then the second series of six exercises is carried out again.

b. Another way is to increase the number of sets on each exercise before moving to the next exercise – for example two sets of ten reps on half squats, with a short rest between, followed by two sets of ten reps on the press-on bench. In due course an increase to three sets on each exercise could be made before moving on to the next exercise.

c. A third form of progression in this programme is to increase the number of reps. For example, an exercise is first carried out with a load that barely permits the completion of ten reps, but as strength is gained the number of reps possible will rise to perhaps 15. At this

117

stage the load is increased by 5 per cent, resulting in the reps possible dropping to ten. When further additional strength is built up, the process is repeated and an increase in load of 5 per cent added again.

Figure 30 gives details of a six-exercise basic weight-training programme using free weights of the bar-bell type. Figure 31 gives details of a 12-exercise basic weight-training programme using dumb-bells, bar-bells and weighted boots or ankle weights. Both programmes aim to improve general fitness and strength.

## A Beginner's Programme

Figure 28 shows a weight-training record card outlining a programme for an unfit beginner. It relates to the six exercises described in the basic weight-training programme shown at figure 30. The programme, which should be supervised, aims to develop the skills of weight training by the gradual application of overload, covering an initial six-week period and exercising three days a week with a rest day between exercise days. Initially only a nominal weight would be used and one set of (perhaps) eight reps carried out during each exercise. The reps are then increased by two every two weeks from eight to twelve reps. As the subject improves in strength, and according to his/her degree of progress, the weight is then increased for the next six-week period. This pattern of training can continue indefinitely.

As further progress is made, it may then be possible for two sets to be carried out on each exercise with the same number of reps but with a short rest between sets. As training continues, changes of exercise will give variation to the programme and avoid boredom.

Figure 28: Weight-Training Record Card

| | | | | WEEKS/REPS | | | | | |
|---|---|---|---|---|---|---|---|---|---|
| EXERCISE | PURPOSE | WEIGHT | SETS | 1 | 2 | 3 | 4 | 5 | 6 |
| Half squats | Mainly for leg and hip strength | Nominal | 1 | 8 | 8 | 10 | 10 | 12 | 12 |
| Press-on bench | To strengthen chest, arms and shoulders | Nominal | 1 | 8 | 8 | 10 | 10 | 12 | 12 |
| Bent forward rowing | For the upper back muscles and elbow flexors | Nominal | 1 | 8 | 8 | 10 | 10 | 12 | 12 |
| Upright rowing | For the shoulders, upper back and elbow flexors | Nominal | 1 | 8 | 8 | 10 | 10 | 12 | 12 |
| Two-hand curl | To develop the biceps | Nominal | 1 | 8 | 8 | 10 | 10 | 12 | 12 |
| Sit-ups (with optional weight on chest) | For the abdominals | Nominal | 1 | 8 | 8 | 10 | 10 | 12 | 12 |

## Weight Training and Sport

Weight training can form an important element of a sports fitness programme. It is a form of training that has values both in promoting general and endurance fitness, and in developing power related to speed. Weight training strengthens muscles and ligaments, so minimising the possibility of joint injury. In the event of injury, it can ensure a more rapid rehabilitation to full playing capacity as well.

Weight training can be used in different ways to achieve different fitness objectives. Resistance training that permits ten to twelve repetitions or so will make for improved strength and fitness. Where lighter weights are used that permit up to 50 repetitions with only short rest pauses between sets, this form of training will lead to improved stamina. Where strength and power are needed, the resistance selected should not permit more than six reps. Effective speed training is dependent on the build-up of strength and power: the participant aims to have a greater power margin in reserve than that demanded by the activity in which he is taking part. These power reserves will enable him to overcome with comparative ease the resistance of the activity he is pursuing – whether it be the power demands required for continuously punting a ball, repeatedly putting the shot or continuously diving to defend his goal.

To summarise, the following effects can be obtained:

119

| IMPROVED STRENGTH | achieved by ten to twelve maximum reps |
|---|---|
| MAXIMUM STRENGTH | achieved by one to six maximum reps |
| POWER | achieved by up to six maximum reps performed at speed |
| STAMINA | achieved by 15 or more maximum reps |

Note that improvement in muscular endurance may accompany the development of strength and be achieved when performing seven to fourteen maximum reps.

WEIGHT-TRAINING EXERCISES FOR SPORT **Many standard weight-training exercises can form an integral part of a preparatory sports fitness training programme.** Standard weight-training exercises will assist the main muscle groups and, dependent on the repetitions applied, promote muscular strength (heavy resistance and a few reps) or endurance (light resistance and high reps). Specific weight-training exercises can relate to the mechanics, anatomy and kinetics of sports or athletic movements. By studying these movements it may be possible to simulate the action (or elements of the action) of the limb or body part involved with a weight-training exercise that develops greater strength throughout the movement. For example, the muscle action and upper limb movements of paddling a kayak can be reproduced in weight exercises (see figure 29); the inclined dumb-bell press[1] simulates the arm action of the shot putter; the declined straight arm pull over[2] follows the pulling arms action of the front crawl swimmer against the resistance of the water. Here, to serve as a brief guide, are some other examples of weight-training exercises that relate to body movements and strength requirements in various sports:

---

[1] Where the subject lies head up on a bench, supported at 45°, and presses vertically.

[2] Where the subject lies head down, feet held by a strap on a bench, supported at 45°, and repeatedly pulls the dumb-bell in an arc from above his head to the vertical.

| SPORT/EVENT | EXERCISES |
|---|---|
| Archery | Dumb-bell press, single-arm rowing |
| Badminton, tennis, squash | Arm lateral raise lying, lunges, single arm rowing |
| Boxing | Inclined alternate dumb-bell press, press on bench, single-arm rowing |
| Canoeing | Alternate dumb-bell press lying, press on bench, single-arm rowing |
| Cycling | Half squats, squat jumps, step-ups with weights |
| Fencing | Lunges, dumb-bell, press lying |
| Shot | Dumb-bell press lying, press on bench, press on inclined bench |
| Sprinting | Half squats, squat jumps, step-ups with weights |
| Javelin | Bent-arm pull over, straight-arm pull over, press on bench |
| Swimming | Declined straight-arm pull over, arm lateral raise lying |
| Major team games | General arm, shoulder, trunk and leg weight exercises |
| Volleyball, basketball | Squat jumps, step-ups with weights, dumb-bell press, straight-arm pull over |

Figure 29: The Action of Kayak Paddling Related to Weight-Training Exercises

THE RELAXED PADDLING ACTION COMPRISES A SIMULTANEOUS PUSH WITH THE UPPER ARM, WHICH IS FULLY EXTENDED, AND THE PULL OF THE LOWER ARM ALLOWING THE PADDLE TO PIVOT AROUND AN IMAGINARY POINT IN FRONT OF THE CANOEIST. FIGURES A AND B SHOW WEIGHT-TRAINING EXERCISES THAT DEVELOP THE MUSCLES WHICH EXTEND AND FLEX THE ARMS.

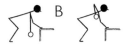

A

PRESS ON BENCH

B

SINGLE-ARM ROWING

Equipment: Bar-bells and weights, bench, bar-bell stands.

Exercise 1: Half Squats

Mainly for hip and leg power. With bar-bell behind the neck, feet comfortably apart, heels raised about one inch on a solid block, breathe out as you bend the knees until the thighs are almost parallel with the floor but keep the back straight. Push up to straighten the legs, breathing in at the same time. Bar-bell stands should be used when progressing to a heavier weight.

Exercise 2: Press on Bench

For chest, arms and shoulders. Begin with your back lying on the bench, bar resting on your chest, hands a shoulder's width apart with forearms vertical. Press the bar to arm's length, breathing in as you do so. Lower under control, breathing out at the same time. When progressing to using heavier weights it is *essential* to use two assistants to position and then remove the bar.

Figure 30: Six-Exercise Basic Weight-Training Programme

| 1 HALF SQUATS | 2 PRESS ON BENCH | 3 BENT-FORWARD ROWING |

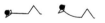

| 4 UPRIGHT ROWING | 5 TWO-HAND CURL | 6 SIT-UPS (BENT-KNEE CURL) |

### Exercise 3: Bent-Forward Rowing

For the upper back and elbow flexors. Lean forward, head up, back flat, knees slightly bent, feet well apart. With hands wider than shoulder width and elbows raised sideways, pull up the weight from the floor to the chest, breathing in at the same time, then lower, breathing out.

### Exercise 4: Upright Rowing

For the shoulders, upper back and elbow flexors. With feet just apart, pick up the bar and hold it at arm's length against the thighs, with knuckles about eight inches apart and facing the front. Pull the bar up by raising the elbows until it is chin height, breathing in at the same time. Lower the bar, breathing out as you do so.

### Exercise 5: Two-Hand Curl

For the upper arm (biceps). With feet apart and arms straight, grip the bar with under-grip and hold it against the thighs with your hands a shoulder's width apart. 'Curl' the weight by bending the arms strongly at the elbows – but keeping the bar close to the body – until the bar rests on the chest, breathing in at the same time. Lower the bar as you breathe out. Let the arms do the work, not your back, and keep the body vertical.

### Exercise 6: Sit-ups (Bent-Knee Curl)

For the abdominal muscles. Lie on your back with hands placed at the side of the head, elbows out, knees bent and feet anchored. Breathing out, raise the head off the floor first, then the shoulders and finally the back. Breathe in as you return under control to the starting position. The exercise can be made more difficult by clasping a weight to the chest.

Equipment: Dumb-bells, bar-bells, weighted boots or ankle weights, medicine ball, bench and bar-bell stands.

### Exercise 1: Half Squats

Mainly for hip and leg power. With bar-bell behind the neck, feet comfortably apart, heels raised about one inch on a solid block, breathe out as you bend the knees until the thighs are almost parallel with the floor, but keep the back straight. Push up to straighten the legs, breathing in at the same time. Bar-bell stands should be used when progressing to a heavier weight.

### Exercise 2: Lateral Raise Lying

For the chest and shoulder muscles. Begin with your back lying on a narrow bench with feet on the floor, or on the floor with the knees bent. Dumb-bells are held at arm's length vertically over the shoulders. With straight arms, lower the dumb-bells sideways, breathing in at the same time, then out as they are raised to the starting position.

### Exercise 3: Trunk-Forward Bend (Trunk Flexion)

For the lower back, hip and rear of the thigh muscles. With feet apart and the bar resting comfortably behind the neck, bend forward from the hips, breathing out as you do so. Keep the back flat. The knees are bent slightly as the trunk lowers to a position almost horizontal. Breathe in as you return to the starting position. Bar-bell stands should be used when progressing to a heavier weight.

Figure 31: Twelve-Exercise Basic Weight-Training Programme

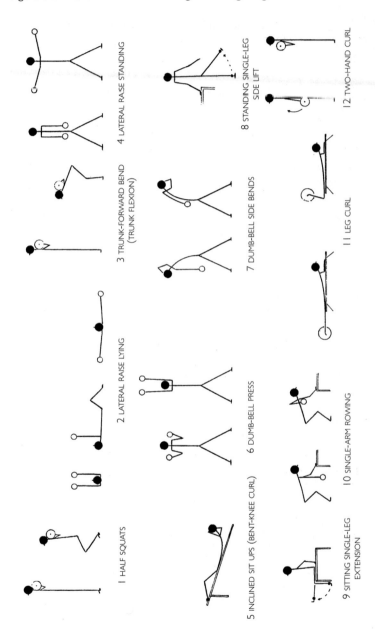

1 HALF SQUATS

2 LATERAL RAISE LYING

3 TRUNK-FORWARD BEND (TRUNK FLEXION)

4 LATERAL RAISE STANDING

5 INCLINED SIT UPS (BENT-KNEE CURL)

6 DUMB-BELL PRESS

7 DUMB-BELL SIDE BENDS

8 STANDING SINGLE-LEG SIDE LIFT

9 SITTING SINGLE-LEG EXTENSION

10 SINGLE-ARM ROWING

11 LEG CURL

12 TWO-HAND CURL

### Exercise 4: Lateral Raise Standing

For the shoulders and upper back muscles. Begin with your feet apart, a dumb-bell held in each hand against the thighs, palms facing inward. Breathe in as you raise the dumb-bells sideways to shoulder height, lifting the chest and head at the same time. Lower, breathing out as you do so.

### Exercise 5: Inclined Sit-ups (Bent-Knee Curl)

For the abdominal muscles. Use an inclined bench, feet supported or held by an ankle strap, knees bent and hands at the side of the head, elbows out. Breathe out as you raise the head off the bench first, then raise the shoulders and finally the back. Breathe in as you lower under control. Note this is a more demanding exercise than the normal sit-ups and can be made even more difficult if a dumb-bell is held to the chest.

### Exercise 6: Dumb-bell Press

For the shoulder, upper back and extensor muscles of the upper arm. With feet apart and a dumb-bell in each hand held at shoulder height, knuckles facing outward, press the dumb-bells fully to arm's length breathing in as you do so and lifting the chest high. Breathe out as the dumb-bells are lowered to the starting position.

### Exercise 7: Dumb-bell Side Bends

For the side of the trunk muscles. Feet apart, grasp a dumb-bell in the right hand, left hand behind the head, then take up the starting position with the body bent to the right but square to the front. Breathing in, bend the body strongly to the left but still facing the front. Do not try to lift the dumb-bell; keep the feet flat on the floor. Breathe out as the starting position is resumed. Repeat the movement five to ten times, then change hands and continue the action while bending to the right.

### Exercise 8: Standing Single-Leg Side Lift

For the abductor hip muscles. Stand with support (e.g. a bench) using weighted boots or ankle weights. With the body weight on one leg, raise the other leg and weights slowly out to the side – keeping the body upright – then slowly lower. Repeat five to ten times, then repeat with the other leg.

### Exercise 9: Sitting Single-Leg Extension

For the thigh muscles. Using weighted boots or leg weights, sit on a bench with legs bent at right angles to the thighs. Extend one leg slowly and fully, breathing in as you do. Breathe out as the weight is lowered. Repeat a number of times, or alternate with the other leg.

### Exercise 10: Single-Arm Rowing

For the upper back, trunk and front muscles of upper arm (biceps). Stand with your feet apart, knees slightly bent, body with straight back supported by your left hand on a bench to the front and left side, right hand holding a dumb-bell vertically below the shoulder. Breathing in, pull up the dumb-bell to a point close to side of the chest. Breathe out as the dumb-bell is lowered to the starting position. After about ten reps, repeat with the other arm.

### Exercise 11: Leg Curl

For the hamstring muscles (back of the thigh). Lie face down on the floor or on a low bench, using weighted boots or keeping a medicine ball griped firmly between the feet. Fully bend the lower legs upwards, pause and then lower to the starting position. Repeat about ten times.

## Exercise 12: Two-Hand Curl

For the upper arm muscles (biceps). With feet apart and arms straight, grip the bar with under-grasp and hold it against the thighs with your hands a shoulder's width apart. 'Curl' the weight by bending the arms strongly at the elbows – but keeping the bar close to the body – until the bar rests on the chest, breathing in at the same time. Lower the bar as you breathe out. Let the arms do the work, not your back. Keep the body vertical.

# SEVEN

# Exercising for Suppleness

Suppleness makes for efficient movement, saves energy and improves performance in skills. It can be defined as the range of movement possible at a joint or series of joints. Suppleness influences posture and movement, giving an indication of general fitness and age. The degree of body flexibility possessed can be influenced by body type and lifestyle.

## LOSS OF FLEXIBILITY

Young children are very flexible. Provided they are given the opportunity and encouragement to participate in healthy recreational exercise and play, this flexibility will continue to increase up to the time of adolescence. After the age of about 15 years there is a natural decrease in flexibility. This decrease is dependent on vocations undertaken, habitual behaviour and the types of exercise practised by the individual. Appropriate regular physical exercise will increase flexibility in all age groups, though the greater increase will be registered by the younger.

The disadvantages of modern lifestyles, being mainly sedentary in nature, are not confined to people of mature age. Loss of flexibility can begin in primary school when children start spending a significant part of their day in fixed positions as they learn. Not many schools have an adequate PE programme to foster the full physical development of children. The lack of what was once active childhood play – which has been brought about by habitually watching television, playing video games and operating computers – does much to exacerbate what for many children can already be a fairly sedentary childhood. Since the body follows the law of use and disuse, in that it must be used regularly and properly if its systems are to be kept in good shape, a sedentary childhood can have its consequences. Organs may not develop fully, or muscles develop their natural power or joints their normal range of movement. So by the time the child is a young adult he/she could also suffer reduced body flexibility, having missed the opportunity to develop to what might have been his/her true physical potential.

Most flexibility problems are caused by changes in the connective tissue around the joint, including the muscles, tendons and ligaments. A degree of suppleness is lost with age as tendons and ligaments thicken, though keeping active and taking suitable exercise can offset this reduction.

Loss of suppleness can be brought about by a number of factors, such as concentrating on one sport or activity. For example, the repetitive action of jogging and cycling can reduce overall body mobility unless followed by general stretching exercises. Poor posture habits are another factor – such as habitually sitting bent over a desk, typewriter or car steering wheel – and may lead to the loss of suppleness in the spine, giving postural problems and round shoulders as the back muscles stretch and the chest muscles shorten. Long periods of sitting can also cause the hamstring muscles to shorten and to tilt the pelvis forward, which affects the angle of the vertebrae in the lower back region and can result in lower back pain. Shortening hamstrings may also lead to 'pulled muscles' that can unexpectedly catch you when sprinting for the bus or reaching to unload a shopping trolley.

Even wearing the wrong kind of shoes can give problems affecting suppleness and posture. For example, soreness in the Achilles tendon can be experienced among people who normally wear shoes with fairly high heels, for if they then walk barefoot or in plimsolls, it imposes a strain on the shortened tendon, resulting in pain and possible rupturing of the tendon's fibres.

It is widely believed that females are more supple than males, although evidence is not conclusive. Females normally have a shorter leg length and a lower centre of gravity. They are therefore able to perform certain movements with more ease than males. However, it is not clear whether any differences in flexibility between the sexes are inevitable or are due to differences in lifestyle.

Suppleness contributes to the avoidance of injury, plus the promotion of good posture that gives psychological benefits, reflecting positive attitudes, thoughts and feelings. Suppleness also helps to ensure a full and enjoyable involvement in sports and pastimes of your choice.

## BASIC FACTORS

There are three factors basic to an understanding of suppleness and flexibility, these are:

ELASTICITY This permits a muscle to stretch beyond its normal resting length and return to that length when the stretching force ceases.

EXTENSIBILITY The maximum length a muscle can be stretched is normally approximately half again its resting length. If a muscle is forced beyond about 60 per cent of its normal resting length its fibres will tear. If the

131

stretching force is excessive, serious damage can be done, for it is possible to pull a tendon (such as the Achilles tendon) from its attachment to the bone.

STRETCH REFLEX When a muscle is stretched, the action is reported along a sensory nerve to the spine and an impulse is sent out along a motor nerve for the muscle to contract automatically (figure 32). This is known as the 'stretch reflex response'. The amount of tension generated in the response varies directly with the rate and amount of movement that causes the muscle to stretch.

The degree of suppleness present or absent affects all-round fitness in several ways:

a. Suppleness determines the possible range of movement in a joint. It is influence by bone structure, the tightness of ligaments, muscle strength and muscle extensibility.

b. Suppleness is specific to each joint. Good ankle flexibility does not necessarily mean good hip or shoulder flexibility. However, a person who can carry out a wide variety of bending, twisting, extending and flexing movements is said to be supple.

c. A lack of suppleness can result in limitations in performance, inefficient technique and, when it comes to speed and dynamic movement, failure to realise true potential.

d. When the range of body movement possible is increased by suitable exercise, greater agility and speed of movement can be achieved and less energy used. Where this flexibility does not exist, the muscles have to work harder to overcome resistance.

e. Suppleness is an important factor in the avoidance of injury, whether from sudden unexpected stress to the body (e.g. a severe twist), distortion (as in a fall), or repetitive exercise that can in due course limit range of movement.

The degree of joint flexibility that we possess is largely inherited, although it can normally be increased, particularly if suppleness training is undertaken before adolescence. The extent of this training can be seen in the remarkable suppleness displayed by some of the young female gymnastic champions.

The components of fitness are best interrelated to give a balanced approach to fitness. Increased flexibility will be of little value unless it is accompanied by increased strength to control the limb action over the range of movement. Additional strength stabilises, controls and even helps protect the joints. On the other hand added strength training can, in some instances, reduce the degree of flexibility that an individual already possesses – unless flexibility exercises are added to the training programme.

Muscles respond to training in two contrasting ways. Firstly, a muscle that is called upon to contract repeatedly will decrease in resting length; on completion of an exercise session the muscle will be shorter. Secondly, a muscle will respond to suitable stretching exercises and actually increase in length. This is effective in combating the condition that sports enthusiasts can sometimes experience after pursuing a set pattern of intensive repetitive exercise. This condition of tight, inextensible muscles – sometimes confused as being 'muscle bound' – can easily be corrected by concluding each training session with a warming-down series of exercises to include gentle but effective stretching exercises.

METHODS OF STRETCHING

Increase in suppleness is achieved by stretching muscles beyond their habitual length. There are two main methods used to increase flexibility, known as 'ballistic' and 'static' stretching.

Ballistic Stretching

Ballistic stretching involves fast movement with the aim of utilising the momentum of the body parts to create a bouncing or jerking action at the end of its normal limit. An example of ballistic exercise is touching your toes with a bouncing action.[1] This type of movement may maintain a range of movement but is unlikely to increase the range for the following reasons:

   a. Unconsciously we only allow sufficient momentum in the movement to permit the limb and associated muscles to go to their present habitual limit of movement.

   b. Sudden jerks applied to a muscle initiates the stretch reflex which will increase muscle tension and only permit a momentary lengthening of the muscle.

   c. Muscle strain may be caused by ballistic stretching resulting in muscle soreness, microscopic tears of the muscle fibres and the formation of scar tissue with some impairment of muscle function.

Figure 32: The Stretch Reflex

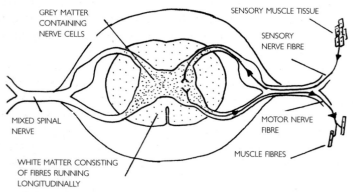

THE STRETCH RELFEX IS THE REFLEX CONTRACTION OF A MUSCLE THAT RESULTS FROM ITS STRETCHING. THE DIAGRAM SHOWS A CROSS-SECTION OF THE SPINAL CORD. WHEN SENSORY TISSUE IN THE MUSCLE IS STIMULATED BY STRETCHING, AN IMPULSE IS CONDUCTED VIA A SENSORY NERVE FIBRE THROUGH A MIXED NERVE TO A JUNCTION WITHIN THE SPINAL CORD. AN IMPULSE IS THEN SENT OUT ALONG THE MIXED NERVE VIA A MOTOR NERVE FIBRE TO THE MUSCLE THAT CONTRACTS THE MUSCLE FIBRES.

[1] Such an exercise, though practised by dancers and gymnasts, is not generally recommended, for the reasons given.

134

Ballistic-type exercises are not recommended for use in general class work, such as step or aerobic dance, due to the wide variation in the participants' fitness levels and age. However, they are favoured by some fitness enthusiasts, dancers and gymnasts. Where used, they should be performed only by the experienced, fit and agile performer with the aim of maintaining mobility.

### Static Stretching

Static stretching involves slow, deliberate movements that take a muscle to the end of its range. The position is then held for a number of seconds, allowing the muscle to adapt to the stretch. In this form of flexibility exercise the stretch reflex, the automatic nervous reaction, is inhibited. There is a slow decrease in muscle tension as the muscle relaxes, permitting a further increase in muscle length and range of movement with no risk of muscle damage. Stretching that involves slow, sustained exercise appears to be the most advantageous. Low intensity stretching, carried out with a raised body temperature, over a duration, can result in permanent lengthening.

Static lengthening can be classified as 'active' and 'passive'. Active stretching involves the performer working alone on flexibility exercises without external aid (see page 145, exercises 4 and 5).

Passive stretching is achieved by external force, usually initiated by another person, while the subject remains inactive. Gravity alone can also be used to assist in passive stretching (see pages 145, exercises 6 and 15). Note that where another person is involved in applying external force to assist a limb into an extreme position, it is *essential* that that person is fully qualified. This type of exercise can, without adequate control, be potentially harmful.

### Training Methods

The following points relate to the development of suppleness, particularly for potential games players and athletes:

a. Cold muscles will resist stretching. If an attempt is made to stretch muscles when cold, strain can be imposed on tendons and ligaments. A thorough warm-up is therefore essential before any flexibility training is attempted. The wearing of suitable warm training clothing will assist the process of warming up. This clothing is best kept on during the stretching exercise session so as to retain the essential high body temperature throughout the session.

b. The initial warm-up should be succeeded by easy stretching, related to each exercise that follows, so as to relax the muscle in preparation for the more serious exercise programme ahead.

c. Stretching exercises should also be carried out while the body is still very warm at the end of the training. This will immediately counter the normal muscle-shortening effects resulting from periods of intense exercise. It is also beneficial to undertake an additional stretching session about an hour later.

d. First of all, isolate the muscle or muscle group to be stretched by placing the joint in the correct position. Static exercise should then be carried out slowly and deliberately. Breathe normally, relax in mind and body and ease into the stretch position. Aim to feel the pull in the belly of the muscle, not at the tendons, and to a point where tension is felt or perhaps some discomfort, but not pain. Hold the stretch position for six to ten seconds to begin with. As the feeling of muscle tension decreases, for the muscle will adapt to the action, stretch a little further. The stretch position held can, over several sessions, be increased from ten to thirty seconds and result in the muscle lengthening. Note that the number of reps to be performed on each exercise should be increased very gradually.

e. Any specific stretching programme could, according to a person's physical condition and requirement, be for a minimum of ten minutes. The frequency depends on how quickly results are required. Three sessions a week could provide a suitable schedule, but one or even two a day would ensure more rapid results.

## Warming-up and Warming-down Stretch Exercises

Following a warm-up, the gentle stretching exercises shown in figure 35 (page 145) are suitable for the average sportsman/sportswoman. These exercises can also be undertaken in the warming-down routine at the conclusion of the exercise session.

### HOW FLEXIBLE ARE YOU? (SEE FIGURE 33)

The following simple tests are aimed at giving the individual an idea as to the degree of flexibility he/she possesses. Some of the tests show how degrees of flexibility can be factually observed and improvements recorded. Before attempting the tests a thorough warm-up should be undertaken. If, when attempting any of the exercises, pain or acute discomfort is experienced, the exercise should be *discontinued*. The exercises should be carried out in a relaxed state, slowly, smoothly and evenly.

### Test 1: Shoulder Pinch

*Object*   To check posture and upper back mobility.
*Method* Stand or sit erect, raise the elbows sideways to shoulder height, then pinch the shoulder blades back together to make a visible crease in your back.

### Test 2: Finger Touch

*Object*   To check arm and shoulder flexibility.
*Method* Place one arm over the shoulder, the other simultaneously behind the back, and attempt to link the fingertips.

### Test 3: Seated Toe Touch

*Object*   To check the flexibility of the lower back and the extensibility of the hamstrings.

Figure 33: Simple Flexibility Tests

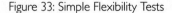

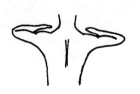

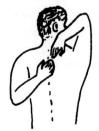

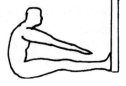

I SHOULDER PINCH

3 SEATED TOE TOUCH

2 FINGER TOUCH

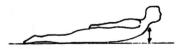

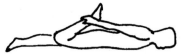

4 BACK EXTENSION

5 KNEE AND THIGH FLEXIBILITY

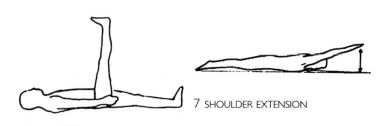

7 SHOULDER EXTENSION

6 HIP FLEXIBILITY

*Method* Sit on the floor with the legs straight, feet against a wall or heavy piece of furniture, hands resting on the knees. Now bend slowly forward to see how far forward you can reach. Do not bounce or jerk into position. Record how far forward you can reach with comfort. If you can reach within four inches of your toes you have reasonable flexibility of the lower back and hamstring muscles. If you can touch your toes your flexibility is good. Note, do *not* attempt this exercise if you suffer from back trouble, or are unfit or overweight.

Test 4: Back Extension

*Object* To check the flexibility of the spine.
*Method* Lie on your front with your hands clasped behind the back, feet fixed. Keeping the chin on the chest raise your head and shoulders from the floor. A partner, with the aid of a piece of string, takes the measurement from the top of the breastbone (the suprasternal notch) vertically to the floor.

Test 5: Knee and Thigh Flexibility

*Object* To check knee flexibility and the extensibility of the thigh muscles.
*Method* Front lying, flex your right knee and grasp the right ankle with the right hand to attempt to touch the buttocks with the heel. Repeat with the left leg.

Test 6: Hip Flexibility

*Object* To check hip flexibility and extensibility of the hamstring muscles.
*Method* Back lying, with one leg straight on the floor, raise the other leg to vertical while also keeping it straight. Then lower it gently. Repeat with the other leg. Do not raise both legs together.

Test 7: Shoulder Extension

*Object* To check shoulder flexibility.
*Method* Lie on your front, chin touching the floor, both arms reaching out straight in front of the shoulders, palms down and together, fingers pointed. Keeping the chin on the floor and arms and wrists straight, raise both arms up as far as possible. With the aid of a partner, measure the vertical distance from the tips of the fingers to the floor. An alternative way to carry out the exercise is to hold a rod horizontally in both hands and measure the vertical distance from the rod to the floor.

For those people who have done little or no exercise, any suppleness exercises planned to help achieve greater body flexibility must be simple and non-taxing. Outlined below are nine simple stretching exercises that can be practised at home. Please first note the following:

a. Though suppleness exercises can serve as part of a warm-up prior to more vigorous training, it is essential that the body is warm before commencing such exercises, for a raised body temperature ensures a greater range of possible movement with less chance of injury. In cool conditions the warm-up can be made more effective if you wear extra clothing and then do some walking, running on the spot or skipping, followed by the suppleness exercises.

b. When you start, carry out the exercise gently, slowly and smoothly.

c. Do each exercise just a few times at first, then gradually build up in later sessions to repeat each exercise, perhaps ten to twelve times.

d. The exercises should be undertaken at least three times a week.

e. Once you feel accustomed to the exercises and your body is becoming more supple, you may feel that after completing the round of nine exercises you would like to repeat with a second round. However, take care that you do not overdo things. Always maintain the gentle, slow and smooth action.

f. If you have experienced trouble with back pain or have any other medical disorder, note the medical precautions on page 61.

Figure 34: Basic Suppleness Exercises

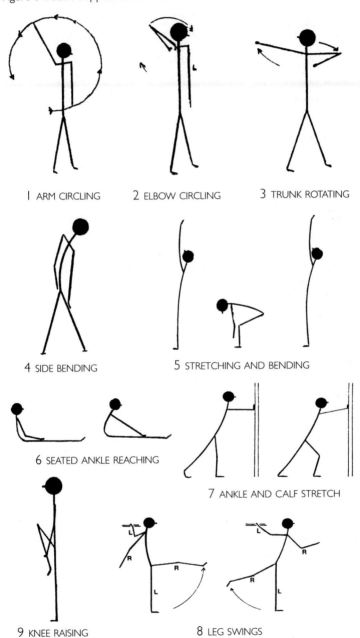

1 ARM CIRCLING   2 ELBOW CIRCLING   3 TRUNK ROTATING

4 SIDE BENDING   5 STRETCHING AND BENDING

6 SEATED ANKLE REACHING   7 ANKLE AND CALF STRETCH

9 KNEE RAISING   8 LEG SWINGS

## Arm and Shoulder Mobility

### Exercise 1: Arm Circling

Stand with feet comfortably apart, arms by the sides. With a straight arm and hips kept facing forward, slowly make a wide backward circle with your right arm brushing your ear and thigh to make the movement as big as possible. Repeat with the left arm. The exercise can be carried out with both arms circling together.

### Exercise 2: Elbow Circling

Stand with the feet comfortably apart. Raise the right elbow up to place the right hand on your shoulder. Rotate the elbow down and forwards, then up and back in a wide circle. Now reverse the action. Repeat with the left elbow, then alternate forwards and backwards.

## Trunk Mobility

### Exercise 3: Trunk Rotating

Stand with feet astride, arms raised sideways to shoulder height. Keeping the feet flat on the floor with the arms held loosely, rotate the trunk gently to the right, then gently to the left. Do not make any jerking or bouncing movement.

### Exercise 4: Side Bending

With feet astride and hands by the sides, keeping the legs straight and body to the front, slowly bend to the left allowing the left hand to slide down your left leg. Do not force or bounce the movement. Return slowly to the upright position, then repeat to the other side and continue.

## Exercise 5: Stretching and Bending

Stand erect and relaxed. Then, raising both arms forward and up, stretch the whole body up as far as you can, fingers pointed. Now, by bending at the hips and knees, slowly lower your hands forward and down towards the floor as far as you can go with comfort. Stretch up and repeat. The movement can, after a while, be made with the arms swinging up on the upward movement and then down behind at the lower position.

## Exercise 6: Seated Ankle Reaching

Sit on the floor with your legs out in front of you as straight as they can be with comfort, hands on top of the thighs. Now slowly and gently reach forward to slide the hands down the legs as far as you can reach. Do not jerk or bounce. Return to the upright position. The exercise will stretch the lower back and also the hamstrings. This exercise should *not* be attempted by anyone with back trouble.

## Ankle and Leg Mobility

### Exercise 7: Ankle and Calf Stretch

Stand at arm's length from a wall with hands placed at shoulder height flat on the wall, fingers pointed upward. Stretch the right leg directly behind you, ball of the foot on the floor, heel raised, toes pointing forward, weight on the left leg. Very gently push the right heel towards the floor, bending the left leg slightly to do so. After several gentle repetitions, change legs.

### Exercise 8: Leg Swings

Stand erect, weight on the left leg, left hand resting on a wall-bar or chair for support. Swing the right leg forward and backward in a smooth rhythmic pendulum action, gradually taking the leg as high forward and as far back as you can with comfort, but keeping the body as upright as possible. Turn around and repeat the exercise with the other leg. The exercise is also good for hip mobility in addition to stretching thigh muscles.

### Exercise 9: Knee Raising

Stand erect. Raise the left knee as high as possible, then grasp the left shin with the left hand and gently pull the leg against the body, keeping the back straight. Lower the foot to the floor. Repeat using alternate legs. If necessary the free hand can hold on to a support. The exercise aims to improve and maintain flexibility of the knees and hips. Note, if you have problems with knees, hips or back, or with balancing, *avoid* this exercise.

### STRETCH EXERCISES FOR INCLUSION IN WARMING-UP AND WARMING-DOWN EXERCISE ROUTINES

These are suitable for sportsmen and sportswomen. Note that before you attempt any stretching exercises the body should be warm, with the aim of eventually gradually increasing the range of body movement.

### Exercise 1: Arm Circling

Make large, relaxed single or double arm circles forward and backward, brushing the ears and thighs.

### Exercise 2: Side Bending

With one arm raised, gently stretch as far as you can go with comfort to each side, allowing the lower hand to slide down the leg as you bend. Then reverse the arms and bend to the opposite side.

Figure 35: Warming-up and Warming-down Stretch Exercises (Suitable for Sportsmen and Sportswomen)

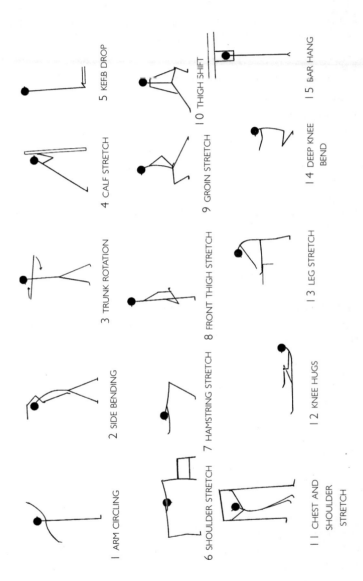

1 ARM CIRCLING
2 SIDE BENDING
3 TRUNK ROTATION
4 CALF STRETCH
5 KNEE DROP
6 SHOULDER STRETCH
7 HAMSTRING STRETCH
8 FRONT THIGH STRETCH
9 GROIN STRETCH
10 THIGH SHIFT
11 CHEST AND SHOULDER STRETCH
12 KNEE HUGS
13 LEG STRETCH
14 DEEP KNEE BEND
15 BAR HANG

### Exercise 3: Trunk Rotation

Keep the feet flat on the floor, arms held loosely at shoulder height, then gently twist to each side. No jerking or bouncing.

### Exercise 4: Calf Stretch

Stand at arm's length from a wall. Slowly bend the arms to lean forward, gently stretching the Achilles tendon and calf muscles.

### Exercise 5: Kerb Drop

Stand supported by the balls of the feet at the edge of a kerb or surface of a similar height, then gently lower the heels to stretch the calves.

### Exercise 6: Shoulder Stretch

With feet apart, hold the top rail of a strong chair, bend the knees slightly, then let the head and chest drop slowly to stretch the shoulders.

### Exercise 7: Hamstring Stretch

With feet apart, keeping the legs straight and back hollow, gently bend forward to feel the backs of the thighs stretching.

### Exercise 8: Front Thigh Stretch

Standing, raise one foot behind, then grasp that instep with the hand to stretch gently the thigh muscles. Keep the knees close together and hips forward. Change to the other leg. (If necessary, to help balance, hold on to a support.)

Exercise 9: Groin Stretch

Place one foot well forward to adopt a front lunge position and gently stretch the groin. Point both feet forward. Reverse the foot and leg positions.

Exercise 10: Thigh Shift

Extend one leg sideways, then bend the opposite knee to stretch gently the inner thigh. Reverse the foot and leg positions.

Exercise 11: Chest and Shoulder Stretch

Using a door frame, reach up to grasp the frame and then lean forward to stretch gently the muscles of the front of the chest and shoulder.

Exercise 12: Knee Hugs

Hug one knee as close as possible to the chest so as to stretch the hamstrings, but keep the other leg straight. Reverse the legs and action.

Exercise 13: Leg Stretch

With one leg raised on a bench or chair, reach forward to grasp the ankle so as to gently stretch the hamstrings. Change legs.

Exercise 14: Deep Knee Bend

With feet together, keeping the heels on the ground, and arms out in front to balance the body, lower yourself to stretch gently the back, hips and ankles.

Exercise 15: Bar Hang

This exercise should be used on the conclusion of the work-out. Hang with over-grasp from a bar to stretch the shoulders and back. (Try 15–30 seconds to start.)

# EIGHT

## Exercising for Speed

- Speed Training
  - Specific Training
  - Categories of Speed
    - Acceleration Speed
    - Sprint Speed
    - Sustained Speed
  - Dependent Components of Speed
  - Speed Training Methods
    - Acceleration Speed Training
    - Sprint Speed Training
    - Sustained Speed Training
  - Speed Drills
    - Arm Speed Practice
    - Leg Speed Practice
    - Standing Start Practice
    - Knee-Lift Practice
    - Speed Variation
    - Acceleration Practice
    - Variation Sprints
  - Developing Optimum Track
  - Sprint Speed

Speed is relative to age. For the very young it is an exciting quality, relished and displayed in joyous darting playground games. For the athletic who are gifted with real pace, the sensation of speed derived from the wind on your face and through your hair – as you sprint for sheer fun along the edge of the tide or dash for the rugby corner flag – gives exhilaration, even a degree of headiness. For others it brings the enjoyment of striding over open countryside, making for relaxation of body and mind and giving a sense of freedom.

But speed is not restricted to running. It covers a wide range of fast movement. In everyday life quick reaction and muscular speed are very useful attributes and enable us to make a dash for the train, catch items if they fall off the shelf, swat those elusive mosquitoes, or react quickly at table-tennis. It can also serve us well in an emergency. Where sport is involved, speed is an essential ingredient of good performance.

Speed is defined as the ability to move quickly. It can also be expressed as the capacity to perform successive movements of the same type at a fast rate – such as the rapid muscular movements, involving many muscle groups, that is required in sprinting; or lesser demanding movements involving specific parts of the body, such as when typing. Individuals may possess specific forms of speed that bear little relationship to other forms of speed required in other sports. For example, the ability to sprint on the track differs from that which is used to sprint cycle, speed skate or make a fast ball throw. This is because many sports require the use of different muscle groups and individuals rarely have the ability to excel in a wide variety of 'fast' sports.

The possession or absence of speed is dependent on a number of factors. Body type has a significant bearing and in adults the mesomorphic powerful build is more suited to generating power and pace. Heredity plays a part in determining both body build and muscle fibre type. Individuals who are capable of explosive movements generally have a predominance of fast twitch fibres in their muscles which make for rapid muscular action and fast, quick body movements (see page 37).

Another body feature that influences speed is limb proportion. Muscles act most efficiently through the movement of short levers. Thus short limbs can move more quickly than long ones. In running, short legs will make for strong muscle action and can give considerable accelerative speed. However, at maximum cadence, they cover less ground per stride compared with the length of leg of the true sprinter, with his distinct body type and well-proportioned limbs (though there are exceptions and some extremely fast smaller sprinters). Different sports and activities – e.g. sprinting, high jumping, shot-putting and as varying as table-tennis and fencing – require their own degree of speed and patterns of movement calling for a high degree of specific skill. But what is important is that speed training can normally improve the performance of the slowest player. For some individuals the improvement can be dramatic.

## SPEED TRAINING

The main trainable aspects of speed are in the areas of style, reaction time and technique. The nature and function of speed varies according to the sport involved. Arm speed is critical to the fast bowler in cricket, the javelin thrower and the sprint canoeist. Leg speed is critical to the football and hockey forward, also the rugby wing. But some sports, such as basketball and tennis, call for both arm and leg speed.

Reaction time is the period that elapses between a stimulus (auditory, visual or tactile) and the muscular contractions made in response. The auditory stimulus can take many forms, from the warning screech of a car's brakes to the crack of the starter's gun. Visual stimulus can be the sudden fast tennis service; or shown in the reaction to the danger of a falling slate. Tactile stimuli include the peak tension felt on the bowstring when an arrow is fully drawn, or the absorbing flexion of a skier's legs and body in response to the pressure experienced in a tight slalom turn. Reaction time can be impaired by fatigue, worry, mental excitement and distraction. Reaction time can be improved with practice provided that the conditions relate to, or simulate, the activity.

Generally, where sport and games are concerned, the initial body position adopted will influence the speed and efficiency of response to a signal. This is seen in the flexed start of the position taken up by the racing swimmer and the crouched start of the 100-metre runner. When a quick reaction is required from a standing position the body weight should be distributed evenly over both feet, heels raised, knees and hips slightly bent, trunk leaning slightly forward with bent arms partially raised. The position is one of alertness. Where rules permit, constant small rhythmical

151

bounce-like movements will stimulate muscle tension in preparation for a fast muscular response. This form of preparatory response is demonstrated when receiving at tennis; or seen in the boxer's constant nimble arm and leg work, aiming to enhance the effectiveness of his punching and deflective defence actions.

## Specific Training

Where an optimum performance is required of a player performing in a set playing position, speed training must be specific and relate directly to the speed skills that the player will require in his position. The attributes of the first-class rugby wing three-quarter are not limited to the possession of blistering speed and determination. They also cover the ability to change pace; effect a lightning side-step off both feet; attack with explosive power; and recover quickly from the prone position after tackling or being tackled ready for immediate counter attack – all aspects of speed play. Training for the wing three-quarter therefore needs to be aimed at the individual elements of speed play involved. For example, specific skill training would be given to the sub-skill and technique of side-stepping, performed fairly slowly at first, then speed training introduced to the skill with the movement practised at increasing pace.

## Categories of Speed

Running speed is determined by stride cadence and stride length. In the open field of play, as offered in the major sports of football, hockey and rugby, speed can be identified in three basic forms.

> ACCELERATION SPEED In games situations it is often necessary to pick up speed very quickly from a standing start. In order to do so, dynamic leg and arm work is required, and much ground contact also made, as the initial transitional strides though fast are comparatively small

so as to generate forward momentum. In this type of running the distance covered may be only 25–30 yards, but the technique provides the acceleration needed to take a football at speed, or defend against a sudden attack. Many players rely on this attribute and are descibed as being 'quick'. They can be very effective even though they may not possess the true sprinting ability to cover the field at high speed.

SPRINT SPEED At times a player may be required to cover 60–80 yards at full pace, perhaps in an all-out attack or defence situation. Once initial speed has been achieved, ground contact is reduced with the increase in stride and sustained leg cadence. Here the technique of the sprinter comes into his own. The knee lift is high, the arm action relaxed and the facial muscles too; the whole action is balanced and harmonious, ensuring a maximum output of sheer pace.

SUSTAINED SPEED A fast, mobile game demands that a player has the capability of performing repeated short-distance sprints to meet the demands of high activity chains of play. For instance, a back in rugby football may sprint to attempt to score; but when tackled, with ball possession lost, he may need to cover a counter-attack, tackle and follow up a kick ahead, then cover the opponents' quick drop-out and so on. An element of endurance training directly related to speed work is therefore of considerable importance. Such training will also help ensure that the level of skill possessed by a player will be retained and not be quickly eroded by the onset of fatigue. In addition, it should be noted that players are often required to keep covering the pitch at cruising speed. The higher the player's sprint speed, the higher will be his cruising speed.

Perhaps the three elements of speed, i.e. acceleration, sprint and sustained speed, have never been more dramatically demonstrated on the playing field than by the 1948 Olympic 4x100-metre relay silver medallist K.J. Jones, the Newport, Wales and Great Britain rugby wing three-quarter. Ken was a rare example of an Olympic athlete who could transfer his sprinting ability on to the pitch: he utilised his blistering acceleration and balanced high-speed running; and combined devastating pace with great determination, both in attack and defence. It was my privilege as a youth to have competed against this gifted, yet so modest, outstanding sportsman.

## Dependent Components of Speed

The development of speed is closely related to the presence of high levels of strength, flexibility and muscular stamina. Muscular strength is essential to the attainment of optimum speed. Suppleness is also important, since this factor influences the range of movement through which force can be applied. Muscular stamina will ensure that speed can be sustained and repeated over a period of time.

In sport dynamic speed can be observed in a variety of forms, such as the sudden dive demanded of a goalkeeper, or the vertical jump of the basketball player to score a basket. The possession of this explosive force is also vital to success in many other sports activities such as ground agility gymnastics (including bounding and bouncing actions leading into forms of somersaults) and athletic events such as triple jumping and shot-putting. The power demonstrated is a composite of strength (muscular force) times speed (rate of muscular contraction).

Such explosive power can be improved by what has become known as 'plyometric training', which involves rebound movements. In simple terms, the principle behind this form of training is quick recoil. It is based on the fact that maximum tension develops within a muscle when it is stretched quickly. The faster the muscle is made to lengthen, the greater is the tension response. For the legs this reaction can be obtained by rebound movements such as squat jumps, single- and double-leg hopping, knee tucks and double-leg bounding. For the upper body, training can take the form of repeated press-ups with a clap, 'explosive' press-ups and dynamic bench presses. In this type of continuous training, exercises should be carried out emphasising speed of movement and consistency in both form and the maximum force used (see figure 36, page 159 for examples of plyometric exercises related to the development of leg speed).

Take note that plyometric exercises are very intensive and pose stress on ligaments and tendons, giving a greater possibility of injury. It is therefore advisable to carry out strengthening basic weight training for *at least six months* before incorporating plyometrics into a training routine.

Speed Training Methods

Interval training can be used in the preparation of participants for track, swimming and power-strength events at all levels by improving muscular strength, speed, muscular endurance and tolerance to oxygen debt. Repetition sprints form the basis of sprint training. When used to develop pure speed, sufficient recovery time must be allowed between sprints to maintain good technique. When used to develop endurance speed, once technique and sprint pace is established, the reps or sets could be increased; or less recovery time could be permitted between sets, but not at the expense of good form.

Training applicable to field games for the three categories of speed (acceleration, sprint and sustained speed) can be divided into, firstly, pre-seasonal training; and, secondly, support training that would accompany seasonal games participation, but is carried out periodically as an alternative to actual sprint work. Pre-seasonal and support training could involve weight training with weights that allow up to ten or twelve reps to develop body and leg strength. It could include plyometrics to give power. Additionally, where sustained speed is required, it could take in circuit training. But it should be noted that the overall effectiveness of sprint training can be reduced if support and sprint training is practised simultaneously. Some suitable training methods for the three categories of speed are as follows:

ACCELERATION SPEED TRAINING Practising for acceleration could include uphill sprints, to build up leg strength and develop a good arm action, and down-slope running to develop leg speed. Actual sprinting on the flat could initially comprise four sets of three sprints of 25–30 yards from a standing start (with adequate recovery periods between sets). Progression can be made by gradually increasing sets and repetitive sprints, always with sufficient recovery periods.

SPRINT SPEED TRAINING Sprint practice must focus attention on correct technique with adequate recovery periods between sprints to ensure continuous quality running. Sprint training could be undertaken over some 60–80 yards at 90–100 per cent effort, with a slow walk back to the starting point. Training may initially comprise three sets each of three reps, with a recovery period of several minutes between reps, perhaps increasing to sets of four and five, but always with adequate recovery between reps and sets.

SUSTAINED SPEED TRAINING Sustained or endurance speed is the quality that enables a player to repeat bursts of speed and sustain fast play. Once good sprinting form and pace are achieved, progressive increase in the intensity of the workload is made by increasing the sprint intervals and reducing the recovery periods. This will eventually bring about a tolerance to the demands of overload and realise the physiological changes that give both aerobic and anaerobic benefits – so developing a player's ability to make repeated sprints to meet the demands of high-speed chains of play without experiencing undue fatigue. Commence with sprints of three sets of three reps over 50–60 yards at 80–90 per cent effort, initially walking back to the start point after each run. Take an adequate rest interval, about four or five minutes, between sets. Progression can be made by increasing the number of reps per set to four then five, or increasing the number of sets to perhaps six or more, or reducing the recovery time. However, quality running must always be maintained.

## Speed Drills

Speed drills can form the basis of a team or individual training programme. The main aim of the drills is to develop good running technique, resulting in efficient movement, energy conservation and greater pace. The benefits of increased pace are not confined to team players or athletes. Anyone can improve his/her running speed and enjoy the achievements of doing so. The surface best suited for training is an open grass area or a running track, suitably pre-measured and marked with flags or cones to denote various sprint distances. Basic speed drills may take the following forms:

ARM SPEED PRACTICE Stand with the feet astride, leaning slightly forward from the hips, head raised. Practise the dynamic but relaxed pendulum arm action, made with the hands raised no further than shoulder height in the forward swing, then back no further than the hip on the backward swing. Gradually increase the arm speed to simulate sprinting, but keep the neck and face muscles relaxed.

LEG SPEED PRACTICE Run on the spot on the balls of the feet, lifting the knees high and accentuating the arm action with shoulders slightly hunched. Gradually increase the speed to sprinting pace.

STANDING START PRACTICE From a standing position the player drives forward, body well angled and initially with rapid transitional strides assisted by a powerful driving arm action. The strides are gradually lengthened as sprint speed is attained at 25–30 yards. The strides are then eased and the exercise repeated.

KNEE-LIFT PRACTICE The player jogs initially with a high knee action. An alternative practice is to pick up speed, then lift the knees to make a high knee sprint over 20–25 yards.

SPEED VARIATION The ability to change speed can be used to wrong-foot a defender. Training can take the form of sprinting at about 90 per cent of maximum effort for 20 yards, coasting at a slightly reduced speed for about 15 yards, then making a sudden all-out acceleration to sprint 20 yards at full power.

ACCELERATION PRACTICE Practice involve gradually picking up speed to make a rolling start, then using a dynamic arm action to build up to near sprinting pace for some 25 yards with good form emphasised. Then slow to a jog or walk before repeating the procedure. If this is used in team practice, it is a good idea to divide the team into ability groups and to place a faster runner in each group to act as a pace-setter.

VARIATION SPRINTS Variation sprints follow the principle of fartlek running, with high activity periods of various lengths interspersed with periods of relaxed jogging or even walking. You may accelerate from a rolling start to sprint 30 yards, slow to jog 50 yards, accelerate again for 50 yards, then walk 150 yards. To achieve progression, work to sets of reps and, when ready, increase the number of reps and sets involved.

Speed drills, in one form or another, have been around for some time. W.G. George (1858–1943), the 'Wiltshire Wonder' from Calne, was a remarkable all-round athlete. A talented footballer and keen cyclist who, it was reported, attained 'alarming' speeds on his cumbersome penny-farthing, he turned to athletics at the age of 19 and was a member of Moseley Harriers. George invented the '100 Up' exercises which consisted of running on the spot and picking your knees up so high as to touch your outstretched palms. In 1885 he ran the mile in 4 minutes 10.2 seconds. For 46 years no man in the world ran faster. His performance was all the more amazing as he suffered from asthma.

## Developing Optimum Track Sprint Speed

The basic principle employed in the quest for optimum track sprint speed is that of overload. This is applied in the form of overstress over a shorter distance than would be performed in competition, but varied with over-distance sprints every two or three training sessions where the athlete would train over a longer distance than is to be run in competition. Take, for example, a club sprinter who wishes to improve his 100-metre performance from 11.8 seconds to a target time of 11.4 seconds. In practice he could run half the distance (i.e. 50

Figure 36: Repetitve Power Training (Plyometric) Exercises for Leg Speed

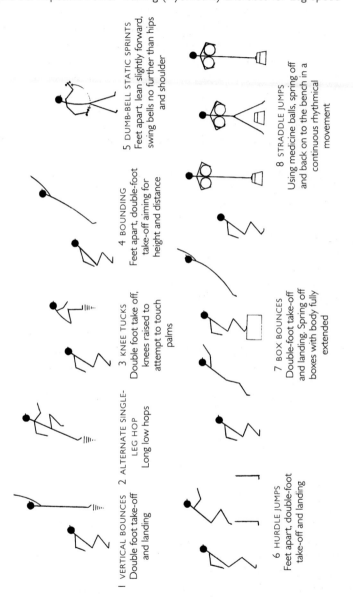

I VERTICAL BOUNCES
Double foot take-off
and landing

2 ALTERNATE SINGLE-
LEG HOP
Long low hops

3 KNEE TUCKS
Double foot take off,
knees raised to
attempt to touch
palms

4 BOUNDING
Feet apart, double-foot
take-off aiming for
height and distance

5 DUMB-BELL STATIC SPRINTS
Feet apart, lean slightly forward,
swing bells no further than hips
and shoulder

6 HURDLE JUMPS
Feet apart, double-foot
take-off and landing

7 BOX BOUNCES
Double-foot take-off
and landing. Spring off
boxes with body fully
extended

8 STRADDLE JUMPS
Using medicine balls, spring off
and back on to the bench in a
continuous rhythmical
movement

metres) all out at half his target time for the 100 metres (i.e. 5.7 seconds), so intensifying the work interval. The workload could initially comprise three sets of two to three repetition sprints. This might be gradually increased to four, then five reps per set, always with sufficient rest between sprints and sets to tolerate the demands of the high intensity effort involved. As the training progresses the target time for the 50 metres would be reduced to 5.6–5.5 seconds. The programme could be varied with over-distance sprints of 120–130 metres every two or three training sessions.

Under-distance training seeks to obtain optimum speed through improving reaction time and style by balancing maximum leg cadence with correct stride length. Over-distance runs develop muscular endurance and the ability to sustain sprint speed over the competitive distance to be run. Note that weight and plyometric training should form important elements of preparatory training for sprinting.

Speed in its various forms is a highly trainable aspect of fitness and, as stated, speed training can dramatically improve the performance of most people. Running is natural to some, but others need to practise to develop correct technique. Some years ago Geoffrey Dyson, the national coach of what was then the Amateur Athletic Association, stressed that it is far easier to develop good running technique in the young than to attempt in later life to eliminate faults already established.

# NINE

# Exercising for Skill

- Factors Affecting Learning
  - Learning Conditions
- Learning Skills
  - Establish the Concept
  - Practise the Whole Skill
  - Break Down the Skill
  - Repetitive Training
  - Rhythm and Force
- Practice Sessions
  - Rate of Progress
  - Skills Practice – Variations
    - Multiple Skills Practice
  - Competition
  - Skills Circuits
    - Sports Skills Circuit
    - General Skills Circuit
    - Activity Skills Circuit
- Skills Development – The Young
  - Activities for the Young

Skill concerns the quality of performance in any physical movement or activity. It is a highly trainable aspect of fitness and can be developed through conscious thought and practice. Skill involves the complex interaction of the body's control mechanisms – the brain, nerves and muscles – all working to achieve a specific aim in the most efficient way possible. The learning of skill can be easy for some people, more difficult for others. What is important is that we are able to recognise our strengths and limitations and are also able to identify suitable skills activities that we can enjoy.

Most people wish to be competent in particular skills that demand physical dexterity, whether it be playing the piano, skating or playing a sport. The desire for competency may have nothing to do with competitive success, perhaps just the satisfaction and enjoyment from the achievement of being able to swim several lengths of the pool or to take part in the village badminton club. On the other hand it is important that, if we wish to, the opportunity is available to develop our full potential. To do so requires an understanding of the principles of skills training plus the availability of good coaching and training facilities. It is worth bearing in mind that skill is an aspect of fitness that is least affected by age, so if a high skills level is achieved in one's younger years, this can be of benefit in later life. It could also help to maintain a sound standard of fitness in middle and old age.

## FACTORS AFFECTING LEARNING

The degree of skill that we can achieve is dependent on a combination of two factors – innate ability and suitable practice. These can be influenced in a number of ways. Your body type, personal attitude, physical condition and present skills level can affect the learning process.

Build, or body type, can make the individual a potentially better player in one particular sport than in another. The lean angular ectomorph would be far more likely to excel at cross-country running than the well-built mesomorph who may be more suited to playing rugby. Differences in temperament can make one person prefer body contact games while another might prefer less boisterous activities. Your readiness to learn a skill, and your degree of physical preparation, will also determine how quickly and effectively the skill is assimilated.

Though a person's learning potential and physical ability may be limited, new interesting training experiences which are administered through well-planned and enjoyable practice sessions can result in high motivation, added interest and therefore greater skills assimilation. The capability and experience of the coach/teacher plays a very important part in realising the attainment of a person's potential. The best results are obtained where a performer possesses a suitable body type for the activity undertaken, is well motivated, has good instruction, possesses set objectives and is prepared to respond to a major challenge.

## Learning Conditions

To be effective, training for skill needs to fulfil a number of conditions. Training must be sufficient and also specific. Training and practice in one skill may have little carry-over to another, for each particular skill has its own specific characteristics – both in type and quality of movement. Though some games have a superficial similarity, the transfer of skills from one sport to another is rarely possible. Badminton and tennis could be expected to have a fair degree of transferability, but the different demands as to positional  play and speed requirements are conflicting. So are the racket strokes, for the heavier tennis racket requires a swinging action whereas the lighter badminton racket is flicked. Each game usually needs a separate approach in skills training and any attempt to obtain simultaneous proficiency in two games may not be feasible in time and effort. The most effective form of skills training is achieved by the rehearsal of the actual skill itself.

When concentrating on learning a skill, use of the right equipment is important. For example, it can be a mistake to practise with a heavier tennis racket or canoe paddle in the belief that the increase in weight will improve skill and handling ability as well as strength. The result could be a deterioration in skill, timing and overall technique.

## LEARNING SKILLS

When a complicated skill is attempted, the individual's performance can at first be awkward and require maximum concentration. Following suitable practice the skill may be performed more easily and call for less effort, both physically and mentally. It would therefore be appropriate to look at how skills are best learnt; the forms of practice possible; and the way in which the body applies skills learnt with little conscious effort. The learning of a complicated skill can be divided into three phases:

ESTABLISH THE CONCEPT First of all, it is important when learning a new skill that the whole skill is demonstrated so that you know what it looks like. This can be done by watching a demonstration by an instructor or good performer, watching a video or film, or studying posters or descriptive drawings.

PRACTISE THE WHOLE SKILL After you have established the basic principles of the skill you should attempt the skill, ideally under the guidance of a coach or instructor. This initial practice will allow you to get a better understanding of what is required, realise your own ability, retain and stimulate your interest further and, from understanding what is required, correct and improve technique.

BREAK DOWN THE SKILL If you find no difficulty with performing the skill you should continue to practise playing particular attention to good form. However, if difficulty is experienced and the activity is too complex to master all at once, the activity should, if possible, be broken down into complete parts or sub-skills. These sub-skills need to be complete in themselves. For example, the breaststroke in swimming can be broken down into parts by practising firstly the arm action; then the arm action combined with correct breathing; then the leg action. Finally the parts are put together and practised as the complete stroke.

## Repetitive Training

Games and activities are made up of many skills, some more complex than others. The skills required by the soccer centre-forward to score goals, or the goalkeeper to defend his goal, must provide an immediate and accurate response to vital game situations. Performance in such skills can be improved by repetitive training where the player is forced to concentrate his attention and effort to deal with repeated similar situations. For example, the football striker may have ball after ball rolled just ahead for him to shoot at goal on the run; or the goalkeeper may be bombarded with shots from set angles that, after a while, would be changed. This is known as 'pressure training' and can be adapted for most sports.

In the initial stages of such training, conscious thought is being used to deal with situations. However, this form of training is based on the fact that once you have learnt a skill the need for fine concentration lessens and the skill becomes a reflex response being made without conscious effort. In simple terms, pressure training helps groove a pattern of movement in the central nervous system that becomes second nature to the performer. This allows freedom to concentrate on the strategy of play. For example, the centre-forward should not need to think of the position of his non-kicking foot as he shoots for goal, nor should the rugby place kicker as he takes a penalty kick.

The reflex action learnt can be further adjusted by the brain from sensory stimuli. For example, a batsman may make an automatic forward drive but adjust his stroke in response to his split-second visual interpretation of the spin and speed of the incoming ball. Once a skill has been learnt the pattern of the movement becomes fixed in your memory, whether it be riding a bike, typing or skateboarding. Even after a long period where practise of the skill has not been possible you can normally, and without much difficulty, regain competence in the activity.

The very great importance of practising correct technique throughout all phases of repetitive training cannot be emphasised too strongly. Without doubt practice makes permanent. The old saying, that practice makes perfect, will only apply if correct technique is always practised in training sessions resulting in poise, balance and perfection of movement.

Suitable rhythm can help improve skills performance. For example, typewriting skills are frequently taught accompanied by music of appropriate rhythm and speed. Once the students have perfected their basic typing skills at an initial speed, the rhythm is gradually but carefully increased to a faster cadence, ensuring that the typing speed is built up without detriment to accuracy. Background music can also help output in a factory, particularly if the music can be linked to the speed of workers' tasks. Aerobic dance classes rely on rhythmic movement linked to music, which motivates and also helps class members to keep time.

All movements have some form of rhythmic pattern. Some are well defined, as shown in the steps of the dancer, the stride pattern between the hurdles of the hurdler, the action of the hammer thrower, or the continuous rhythmic action of the crawl swimmer giving a constant beat of – pull (arms), kick, kick, kick (legs). When you are learning a skill, such as serving in tennis, the actions form a rhythmic pattern involving the compilation of force: the back-and-forward swing or movement, the culmination of force (the delivery) and the dissipation of force (the follow-through). Each element of the pattern is critical to the achievement of correct technique.

When watching a demonstration, think the activity through carefully. Note the whole movement, the time intervals and degree of force that is applied to the different portions of the movement, the point of culmination of effort, then the dissipation of force. Now practise the skill. Perhaps you are learning to bowl on the green. Make the back swing, then the forward swing, the compilation of force, followed by the delivery (the force culmination) then finally the follow-through (the dissipation of force). If possible, check your technique on a video or in a mirror. Figure 37 shows the application of force to the skills of golf, bowling, athletics (javelin and discus), cricket and tennis.

## Figure 37: Aspects of Movement – Application of Force

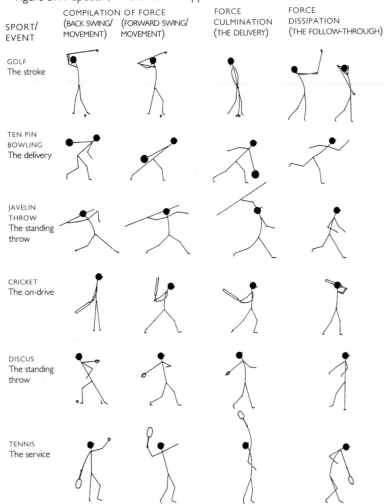

| SPORT/ EVENT | COMPILATION OF FORCE (BACK SWING/ MOVEMENT) | (FORWARD SWING/ MOVEMENT) | FORCE CULMINATION (THE DELIVERY) | FORCE DISSIPATION (THE FOLLOW-THROUGH) |
|---|---|---|---|---|
| GOLF The stroke | | | | |
| TEN PIN BOWLING The delivery | | | | |
| JAVELIN THROW The standing throw | | | | |
| CRICKET The on-drive | | | | |
| DISCUS The standing throw | | | | |
| TENNIS The service | | | | |

## PRACTICE SESSIONS

The length of practice sessions is significant. They should not last too long, for if they do they will result in loss of concentration, incorrect performance being rehearsed and the wrong technique learnt. Fairly short practice sessions that are

167

followed by reasonable rest intervals are generally more effective than long practice sessions with short rest intervals.

## Rate of Progress

In the early stages of skills training progress can be rapid. This is generally followed by a slowing or levelling off of the learning process.

Plateaux in learning can occur because:

a. The skill is too complex and needs to be broken down into simple movements to be practised individually, before practising as a whole.
b. Training sessions have been too long or too intense, or rest intervals are too short.
c. Training has become monotonous and needs to be more varied.
d. Personal achievement levels have been reached.
e. Tiredness is affecting your performance.

Do not merely go through the motions of practising, but practise with feeling and concentration. Think the activity through and, if necessary, analyse your movements so that you know what is correct or incorrect.

## Skills Practice – Variations

Skills practice needs to be interesting and effective. The following variations aim to provide motivation and enjoyment through personal challenge and competition.

MULTIPLE SKILLS PRACTICE More than one skill can be introduced at a time into a practice with several players working together. For example, in volleyball, players can be called upon to work in threes – one 'serving', one 'setting up' and the third player 'spiking' back to the server. After practising the sequence a number of times, the players change position. Further variety involves combining skills using several players – for example, passing, dribbling and shooting in basketball, with other players defending and blocking. When you are practising parts of a game it is important that, as soon as possible, these parts are applied under actual playing conditions.

COMPETITION The value of competition increases with age from childhood to adulthood. Even in childhood competition gives a reason and stimulus for effort. It concentrates the body both physically and mentally. It also develops the power to endure and to hold on as long as others, or for longer. Competition enlivens practice and can motivate players to give maximum performance in skill as well as physical effort. Competition can take various forms. It can aim to test and develop skill and speed of movement, as with inter-team basketball passing relays, or football or hockey dribbling relays. It can be used to test skills accuracy, such as goal-kicking, netball shooting or tennis serving.

Competition can contribute in the practice of tactics as well. For example, the defensive ability of two footballers can be judged in competition with the attacking skills of three opponents. Competition confirms a standard of achievement, individual or team. However, care needs to be taken so that the demands are suitable for the age, understanding and physical ability of those taking part. If not, the exercise can be counter-productive, resulting in loss of interest and possibly physical strain.

SKILLS CIRCUITS A skills-training circuit aims to improve specific skills through quality repetition. Such circuits can be devised to relate to selected sports, general skills or recreational activities. This type of concentrated training can prove highly effective, being enlivening and having a particular appeal to young people. Though the main aim of the circuit is to develop skill, there can be secondary benefits in improved general fitness.

Like circuit training, a skills circuit involves a number of exercise stations, each being the location of a specific exercise which has been selected for its suitability in developing certain skill(s). The sequence of exercises should

169

be organised to avoid two successive stations laying stress on similar muscle groups, or being too demanding physically. Players are required to practise each skill a set number of times, or for a set time, as decided by the coach/instructor. According to the type of sports and general fitness skills involved, skills circuits can be laid out in a gymnasium, hall or outdoor area – but always under the direction and supervision of a qualified instructor. Examples of three types of skills circuits are given below.

SPORTS SKILLS CIRCUIT Some skills lend themselves to individual practice, but in the example shown of a basic rugby football skills circuit (figure 38) most of the practices require two players or more working together. The range of skills possible will depend on the training facilities being used. For example, much practice can be carried out in a suitably sized indoor area, but most kicking practice (cross-kicks from the wing, punting, screw kicking or place kicking) and practice catching high balls naturally requires the space of a pitch or playing field.

GENERAL SKILLS CIRCUIT A general skills circuit aims to develop co-ordination and body control through the practice of a variety of skills such as ball handling, running, climbing, balancing and jumping. This type of circuit can be particularly suited to children. It provides the opportunity of developing basic skills, initiative and daring. It also helps stimulate an interest in taking part in regular exercise, so contributing to the development of the young. The circuit can be set up in a gymnasium, hall or open space and will give much enjoyment and fun. Figure 39 gives an example of some basic skills that may be included in a supervised general skills circuit. Many of the skills can be adopted for use in an inter-team skills competition.

Note that where there is an element of risk, as with climbing or balancing exercises, close supervision must be given.

ACTIVITY SKILLS CIRCUIT The principles of skills circuits can be adapted to many outdoor activities and can vary from

Figure 38: Skills Development – Basic Rugby Football Skills Circuit

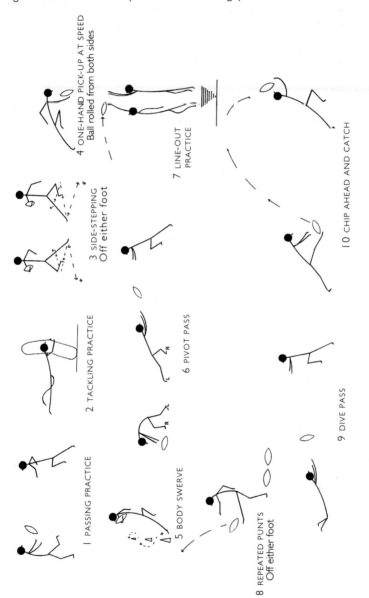

Figure 39: Skills Development – Selection of Basic General Skills for a Children's/Youth Training Circuit

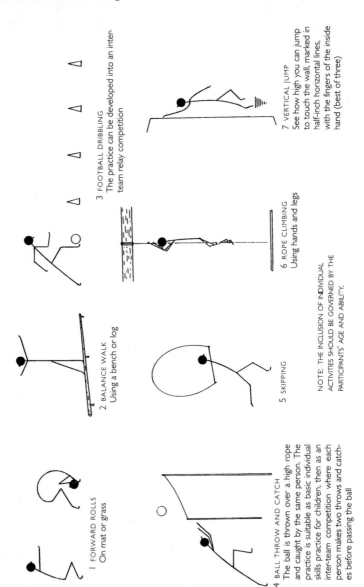

1 FORWARD ROLLS
On mat or grass

2 BALANCE WALK
Using a bench or log

3 FOOTBALL DRIBBLING
The practice can be developed into an inter-team relay competition

4 BALL THROW AND CATCH
The ball is thrown over a high rope and caught by the same person. The practice is suitable as basic individual skills practice for children, then as an inter-team competition where each person makes two throws and catches before passing the ball

5 SKIPPING

6 ROPE CLIMBING
Using hands and legs

7 VERTICAL JUMP
See how high you can jump to touch the wall, marked in half-inch horizontal lines, with the fingers of the inside hand (best of three)

NOTE: THE INCLUSION OF INDIVIDUAL ACTIVITIES SHOULD BE GOVERNED BY THE PARTICIPANTS' AGE AND ABILITY.

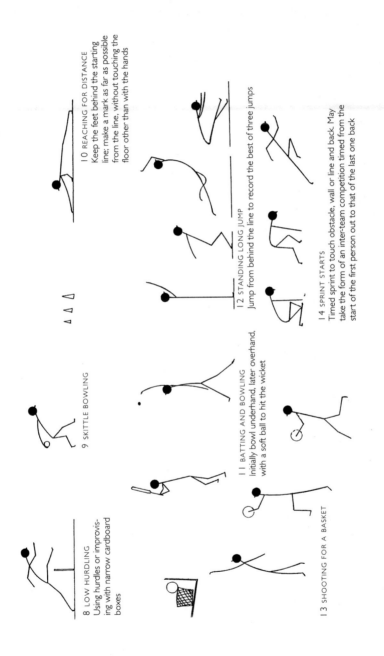

8 LOW HURDLING
Using hurdles or improvising with narrow cardboard boxes

9 SKITTLE BOWLING

10 REACHING FOR DISTANCE
Keep the feet behind the starting line; make a mark as far as possible from the line, without touching the floor other than with the hands

11 BATTING AND BOWLING
Initially bowl underhand, later overhand, with a soft ball to hit the wicket

12 STANDING LONG JUMP
Jump from behind the line to record the best of three jumps

13 SHOOTING FOR A BASKET

14 SPRINT STARTS
Timed sprint to touch obstacle, wall or line and back. May take the form of an inter-team competition timed from the start of the first person out to that of the last one back

Figure 40: Skills Development – Kayak Skills Practice circuit
(Intensified skills training on the river using buoys)

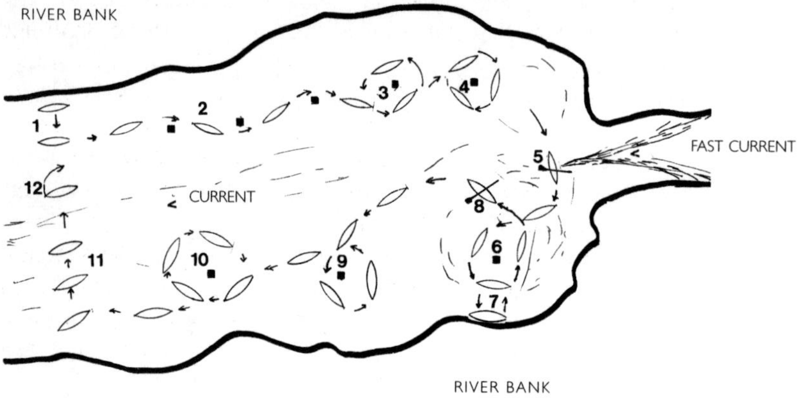

1. DRAW STROKE OUT FROM START POINT ON BANK
2. PADDLE FORWARD USING STERN RUDDER AROUND BUOYS
3. CIRCLE LEFT
4. CIRCLE RIGHT
5. CROSS STRONG CURRENT, LEANING DOWNSTREAM INTO EDDY
6. TURN INTO EDDY
7. SCULLING, DRAW INTO AND OUT FROM BANK
8. ENTER MAIN CURRENT, LEANING DOWNSTREAM
9. USING LOW BRACE (TELEMARK), TURN LEFT
10. USING LOW BRACE (TELEMARK), TURN RIGHT
11. FACING DOWNSTREAM, FERRY GLIDE ACROSS TO START POINT
12. TURN UPSTREAM AND REPEAT CIRCUT

adventure camping and survival skills – such as bivouac making, rope handling, fire laying or emergency stretcher construction – to the dynamic skills required for white-water canoeing. Figure 40 shows how a purposeful kayak skills circut can be set up on a small stretch of river with the use of plastic containers which have been anchored to act as buoys. Such a circuit will ensure maximum pressure-type training practice in a comparatively limited area of water and result in a high degree of skills assimilation.

The fostering of enjoyable active play is important to the physical, mental and social development of children, whether it be undertaken at school or at home. Play is an innate, powerful impulse that in healthy young children enables them to express themselves through physical movement and achievement. The impulse drives them to experiment and to try new ways of doing things, for infancy is a time of exploration, of curiosity through active interest. It is also a time of almost ceaseless energy. However, as a child grows older, the forms of play change and become more complex. As he passes through one stage of growth to another, the play interests continue to change so as to keep pace with the further physical and mental development of the child.

During these early stages the child should first be encouraged to practise basic skills, for example how to pick up a ball and throw it. Later the child should progress to catching the ball; then, at the late infant and junior stage, the child should take part in and contribute to simple team games. In this way the child's physical development can be fostered and skills potential realised. There can be no fine chronological dividing line to mark the changes in developing play interests in children, but there is a broad pattern that can be helpful when considering skills development.

Initially the baby of about one year is mainly interested in himself, though he is aware of other children about him and what they can do. Before long his play and skills performance will become imitative. He will respond to goodbye waves with similar motions and, from observations of adults' action, attempt to pick up the telephone and converse in baby talk. The infant period that follows covers the years of about three to five. This is a time of rapid growth and great emotional change. His play is still individual but gradually play will become imaginative as well as more imitative. He will at the pre-school stage enjoy 'being' an aeroplane, a bunny or a kangaroo. He may soon take part in a simple brief game or race and eventually take his turn in a team. He will also enjoy repetition – particularly the simple games, races and skills which he has been taught and is familiar with – but at this stage he will have

175

little interest in games that have detailed rules. It ought to be noted that infant games should require little sustained attention or physical endurance, but through the medium of encouraged imaginative play there can be the opportunity for the infant to commence finely controlled movements that will, in due course, lead to the promotion of skill.

The junior period of a child's development covers the ages of about five to nine years. Initially, play patterns remain mainly individual; but self-assertion is stronger, so each child should have the opportunity of being, for a brief time, the leader or centre of interest – such as the 'catcher' in a chasing game. As the child grows older, neuro-muscular skill increases so that big balls can be handled with comparative ease. At this stage the child also possesses greater physical agility and determination, which is well demonstrated in dodging games and running 'all out'. From about the age of six years an involvement in mini football and mini rugby, both played to simple skills and rules, can have an appeal. The junior period also sees the commencement of hero worship of sports stars such as footballers and cricketers, and perhaps the desire to identify with the best football teams by wearing their colours.

All these factors can be used to stimulate the child's interest and involvement in active skills practice. However, skills training should be very basic and carried out for short periods with 'activity' being the main theme of any lesson or practice session. As the child gains in play experience, he will develop the capacity to understand very simple tactics, though systematic marking (as in football or netball) can be too difficult for the junior to understand. Games need to be kept simple. Cricket, for example, played by juniors to complex adult rules with periods of inactivity will have little appeal. However, a game of continuous cricket, where there is much activity and where all the children are deeply involved, will have a far greater attraction. This junior period of a child's life sees an increase in attention and also in endurance, so that games and activities planned can be longer than those played in the infant phase.

Generally speaking, from the age of about nine to about eleven years the attitude of the child changes. Competition now has a particular appeal and rivalry plays a part. But competitions for children of this age need to be easily understood and must give a quick result. Now is the time to encourage skills practice such as dribbling footballs around a row of skittles or sticks, building up to an inter-team dribbling competition and then gradually leading to an understanding of positional play and related basic skills.

The formative years of the young are critical to their physical development and can relate to their future health and

Figure 41: Activities and Games for the Young

| ACTIVITY | ACTIVITY |
| --- | --- |
| Agility exercises | Hoop play |
| backward rolls | Hopping |
| cartwheels | Hopscotch |
| forward rolls | Jumping for distance and height |
| hand stands etc. | Jumping jacks |
| head stands | Kite flying |
| Aquatics | Leapfrog |
| diving | Measuring distance, weights and liquids |
| paddling | Model aeroplane flying |
| splashing | Model making |
| swimming | Mountain biking |
| wading | Nature walks |
| Balancing | Obstacle races |
| low bench | Painting pictures |
| one foot | Park walks |
| Ball | Piggy back |
| bouncing | Roller-blading |
| catching | Roller-hockey |
| Bat and ball | Rope skipping |
| Bunny hopping | Relays |
| Camping | Sailing model boats |
| setting up camp | Scooting |
| simple woodcrafts | Skateboarding |
| table setting | Skating |
| Climbing | Skipping |
| apparatus | Snowman building |
| ropes | Swings |
| trees | Tag |
| Cycling | Throw for distance |
| three-wheeler | Tobogganing |
| two-wheeler | Trampolining |
| Drawing | Walking |
| Egg and spoon race | Watering the garden |
| Fishing | 'Wheelbarrow' races |
| Hide and seek | |

happiness. The ultimate aim of skills training for the young should be the achievement of physical vigour and alertness, quick co-ordination of hand and eye, and resource and endurance – all contributing through a continuing involvement in enjoyable habitual exercise to the development of a sound standard of fitness, body development and related bone health.

## Activities for the Young

Some of the activities that can help contribute to the skills and physical development of the young are outlined on the previous page. They include an element of active hobbies as well as recreational pursuits. The activities undertaken would vary according to age, interest and ability of the child. As already stated, where there is an element of risk there must *always* be suitable adult supervision.

# TEN

# Exercising at Home

- Home Exercise and Cross Training
- Home Exercise and Bone Health
- Stationary Walking
- Stationary Running
- Stationary Scout Pace
- Stationary Cycling
- Skipping
- Stair Climbing
- Step-ups
    Step Training
- Home Circuit Training
- Home Weight Training
    Dumb-bell Exercises
    Exercises with Leg Weights or
        Against Resistance
- Isometric Exercises
    Method and Progression
- Conditioning Exercises (Callisthenics)
    Grades
    High Impact Exercises
    Method and Progression
- Aerobic Dancing
- Indoor Training: A Simple Guide to
    Exercise Training Machines
- Home and Multi-gym Training Equipment

Not everyone has the opportunity of using public recreational facilities or those of sports clubs. Many cities and towns lack adequate play areas. In built-up regions there may be few quiet roads or lanes on which to run or cycle, the pavements may be too congested for exercise walking and the parks possibly unsafe. This can pose a problem for those who want to do some positive regular exercise and a common cry can be 'I just do not have a place to exercise'. The solution may lie in what you can do in your own home.

Exercising at home is feasible. Nothing very special or very expensive in the way of equipment is required. Some exercises can be carried out in a reasonably sized room, others can be practised in a garage or on the patio. When practising indoors you are not limited by wet, windy, cold or hot weather conditions. With a little planning the following activities are possible:

| | |
|---|---|
| Stationary walking | Step-ups |
| Stationary running | Home circuit training |
| Stationary scout pace | Home weight training |
| Stationary cycling | Isometric exercises |
| Skipping | Conditioning exercises (callisthenics) |
| Stair climbing | Aerobic dancing |

HOME EXERCISE AND CROSS TRAINING

As with many forms of fitness training, the problem with home exercising is the retention of motivation. Exercising at home needs to be carefully planned to maintain an on-going appeal. Programmes need to be creative and with an element of challenge. From the range of exercise activities possible at home you can devise your own enjoyable 'cross-training' programme, that is, an exercise programme that combines a variety of work-outs to meet *your* fitness interests. A cross-training programme could, for example, include stationary walking followed by an element of conditioning exercise to music and some weight work; then continue with stationary cycling to cover an indicated distance at a set speed; then conclude with a warm-down.

In order to get the most out of your exercising, whether it be at a very modest level or at high intensity, set down aims, record what you do and really enjoy your work-outs.

Much research is being undertaken into the effects of weight-bearing physical activity and the resulting degree of benefit that such exercise has in relation to the promotion and maintenance of bone density. In due course, empirical findings may give fine values of specific activities and exercises in this area. In order to give the home exerciser a *general* guide as to the possible bone health benefits of the various forms of home exercises that follow, estimates are made with a grading of 'high', 'medium' or 'low' according to their possible effect on bone density. These *broad* gradings could be influenced further by changes in the degree of effort that is applied to an activity and also changes to the work duration. For example, stationary running carried out for only very short periods, would not justify a 'medium' assessment. In addition, the *approximate* value of each exercise in terms of stamina, strength and flexibility is given in a 1–4 score (4 being the highest score).

Before you undertake any of the following exercises, refer to the medical precautions on page 61 and get yourself checked out by your physician if necessary. This check is also advisable for those prone to osteoporosis. Note that the benefits of gentle, careful exercise, performed correctly, are considered by the Office of Health Economics to outweigh any associated risks of accident or fracture. However, older people should always be directed to less demanding exercises such as stationary walking and stationary cycling; where weights are used they should be of the lighter variety, where no excessive strain can be put on joints and muscles, and with expert instruction first given.

## STATIONARY WALKING

Bone Health: Low    Stamina: 2    Strength: 1    Flexibility: 1

Stationary walking is a basic activity that will help to maintain general fitness. If carried out with a degree of vigour, it will improve general fitness. It will also help maintain leg and ankle flexibility. You must wear comfortable walking shoes, tennis shoes or trainers.

First of all stand erect, ankles together and toes pointing forward. Now start to walk purposefully on the spot, with the toes still pointed forward and the arms swinging gently in rhythm with each step. Each foot should be raised about four inches. Commence with a comfortable pace and count when each foot touches the floor. Count the number of paces you take in ten seconds, then multiply by six to give your walking speed; 120 steps per minute is a reasonable pace but, if this is too fast or too slow, adjust the pace to suit you. If you are a beginner and dependent on your standard of fitness, commence with a timed walk for perhaps three to five minutes at a comfortable constant pace, then increase the walk by adding one minute every three sessions.

As you become familiar with the exercise, increase your speed and raise the knees higher. If space permits, walk around the room/training area. Additional progress can be made by increasing the length of the training period; by carrying hand weights to 'power walk' (see page 76); or by changing into an easy marching action. The arms are now swung higher and the knees raised further, but avoid crashing the feet down – just place them deliberately with each step. You can also increase the number of times you carry out stationary walking each day. A music tape with the right beat can help maintain a good walking rhythm (see page 232, the use of treadmills).

STATIONARY RUNNING

Bone Health: Medium    Stamina: 2–3    Strength: 1–2
Flexibility: 1–2

Stationary running is a useful basic indoor aerobic exercise. However, it is an exercise that can be hard on the ankles and back, so wear well-cushioned shoes and run on a soft surface such as a mat or carpet, to lessen any shock effect.

To start, stand with the arms hanging loosely at the sides, fingers relaxed and the feet pointing forward. Your running action should be light and easy, with the arms swung low in perfect balance with the action of the legs. The feet should at first be raised no more than about four inches. A beginner requires a stationary running programme that initially imposes little physical demand. Such a programme may commence with the beginner running for only one, two or three minutes, according to his/her basic fitness standard; exercising three or four times a week; then progressing to the next stage at the end of the week (or when ready to do so) by adding 15, 20, 40 or 60 seconds, according to his/her ability. The less fit should run for an even shorter time to start with, then progress by adding ten or fifteen seconds, when they are fit to run for longer.

Time your pace the same way as for stationary walking by counting for ten seconds as each foot touches the floor, then multiplying by six to give your step-per-minute figure; 180 steps per minute is a reasonable pace, but if that is too fast try 150–160 steps per minute. After a while, raise the knees a little higher so as to lift the feet to about eight inches. Some people like to run or walk in time to music. If you have a tape with the right beat it can be enjoyable, while keeping the rhythm going and reducing boredom.

Stationary running can be varied in a number of ways, with progressions introduced according to your ability and fitness:

a. Gradually increase the time run.
b. Vary your running pace with a set number of steps at moderate speed, gradually working up to a faster speed.
c. Introduce several short relaxed 'sprints' into your running programme with the knees lifted high, the body leaning into the sprint and the arms working to balance the leg sprinting action. Then gradually slow down to your normal stationary running pace.
d. After a set number of steps, introduce several burpees or squat jumps (page 218) which will greatly increase the intensity of the exercise and its training effect.
e. After bursts of higher intensity stationary running, if space permits, run slowly in a figure of eight or a circle around the training area before resuming normal stationary running. Figure-of-eight running avoids lateral stress on knees and ankles that can be

encountered if tight circles are run in the same direction.

Figure 42 shows a beginner's ten-week/stage stationary running programme with a constant step-per-minute frequency of your choice and an optional build-up running time from three minutes, adding 20 or 40 or 60 seconds per week/stage.

Figure 42: Beginner's Stationary Running Programme

| WEEK/STAGE | STEPS PER MINUTE (OPTIONAL) | TIME IN MINUTES/SECONDS (OPTIONAL) | | |
|---|---|---|---|---|
| 1 | 140–200 | 3.00 | 3.00 | 3.00 |
| 2 | 140–200 | 3.20 | 3.40 | 4.00 |
| 3 | 140–200 | 3.40 | 4.20 | 5.00 |
| 4 | 140–200 | 4.00 | 5.00 | 6.00 |
| 5 | 140–200 | 4.20 | 5.40 | 7.00 |
| 6 | 140–200 | 4.40 | 6.20 | 8.00 |
| 7 | 140–200 | 5.00 | 7.00 | 9.00 |
| 8 | 140–200 | 5.20 | 7.40 | 10.00 |
| 9 | 140–200 | 5.40 | 8.20 | 11.00 |
| 10 | 140–200 | 6.00 | 9.00 | 12.00 |

Note: Only progress to the next stage when you are ready to do so.

Steps per minute, suggested here as between 140 and 200, can be selected according to the pace you find most comfortable that will allow you to carry out a conversation with a companion, real or imaginary. If you are too breathless to do this, slow down and, if need be, walk for a while. On the other hand fitter people may find the progressions insufficiently demanding, or they may require a longer running period. Therefore make the necessary adjustments. (See also page 232, the use of treadmills.)

**Bone Health: Medium    Stamina: 2–3    Strength: 1–2
Flexibility: 1–2**

Stationary scout pace (see page 76) is a form of moderate aerobic exercise comprising alternate walking and running. Its intensity can be varied according to fitness and age. A beginner could, for example, walk on the spot at a comfortable walking pace for five minutes, raising the foot to about four inches with each step. Count and note your steps per minute. Now break into a stationary run, again at a comfortable pace, for one minute, raising the feet to about eight inches off the ground. Check and note your steps per minute. Repeat the sequence several times Variations and progressions can be made by gradually increasing the running phase and decreasing the walking phase, by altering the speed of both the walking and running phases, and by increasing the number of phases in each exercise session.

**Bone Health: Low–Medium   Stamina: 2–3    Strength: 2
Flexibility: 1**

The stationary cycle is possibly the safest and most efficient type of indoor training equipment. As the body is supported, relatively little stress is placed on the joints. It is therefore an excellent exercise machine for the overweight, the older person and people in rehabilitation programmes, as it assists with the maintenance of general fitness and leg strength. Stationary cycling helps build up aerobic capacity and tone up muscles in the buttocks, hips, thighs and legs. It is generally accepted that the effort required for four miles' cycling equates to the effort of running one mile. Therefore sedate slow cycling is of little value for aerobic fitness, though it does exercise the hip and knee joints. As cycling is a repetitive movement, there is a tendency to lose suppleness, so gentle stretching exercises undertaken after a cycling session can be beneficial.

There are many designs of stationary exercise cycles on the market. Prices can be as high as several hundred pounds for the most complex ones incorporating electronic consoles that monitor speed, distance, time, calories and pulse. However, it is not necessary to spend a lot of money to obtain a machine that can meet the needs of the home-exerciser, but the cycle should have certain features. Firstly, it must incorporate a fully adjustable seat and handlebars. These features are essential to adopt a comfortable position and to avoid damage to joints and muscles. Most of your body weight should be on the seat. The handlebars should be adjusted to allow the rider to lean slightly, but comfortably, forward and not sit bolt upright. The seat must be adjusted so that the legs are almost fully extended when the ball of the foot is at its lowest position on the pedal. Pedalling with the correct seat position allows the legs to act as a powerful lever and also avoids harmful strain on the knee and hip joints if the seat is set too low. Secondly, the minimal instruments required are a speedometer and a distance meter. Some designs may not have these recording features and are of limited value, for it is then difficult to gauge effort and measure progress when carrying out aerobic training programmes.

Many designs have calibrated brake resistance devices to increase or decrease the workload on the rider. It should be noted that, when aiming for aerobic fitness, it is not necessary to strain yourself. The resistance device is therefore initially best set at zero or minimal tension for a beginner, allowing the rider to sustain his effort throughout a session and so benefit aerobically.

Some home-exercisers may be middle aged, with little or no experience of stationary cycling, and may have done little exercise. They therefore need to make a very gentle start. A simple way to do this is first of all to practise at a comfortable speed that will allow you to carry out the talking test (see page 32). If you are too breathless to do so, slow down. Once familiar with the machine, and having discovered a comfortable 'cruising speed', start with an exercise period of three to five minutes' cycling three to four times a week. Add 30–60 seconds each week, or when you feel you are ready to do so.

Those more familiar with stationary or road cycling may

wish to pursue a programme at a higher intensity, cycling twice a day for three or four days per week. The five-week/stage progressive stationary cycling programme (figure 43), aiming to build up cycling fitness, gives an example of a home-exerciser practising at an 'exercise speed' of his/her choice. This is given in the example as 15 mph, building up over five weeks/stages with twice daily sessions that increase from four to twelve minutes. According to ability, if necessary amend the exercise speed to suit you, but only advance to the next stage when you are ready to do so.

Figure 43: Five-Week/Stage Progressive Stationary Cycling Programme

| WEEK/STAGE | TOTAL MINUTES PER DAY | TWO SESSIONS PER DAY (MINUTES) | EXERCISE SPEED (MPH) | MILES PER SESSION | FREQUENCY PER WEEK (DAYS) |
|---|---|---|---|---|---|
| 1 | 8 | 4 | 15 | 1 | 3–4 |
| 2 | 12 | 6 | 15 | 1.5 | 3–4 |
| 3 | 16 | 8 | 15 | 2 | 3–4 |
| 4 | 20 | 10 | 15 | 2.5 | 3–4 |
| 5 | 24 | 12 | 15 | 3 | 3–4 |

Note: If the exercise sessions are increased further, provided they are of sufficient intensity and are carried out for 15 minutes or more per session, aerobic benefits will also be gained.

Dependent on personal fitness levels, either of the two progressive programmes described above can be incorporated into a home-exercise cross-training programme of your choice. (See also page 230.)

SKIPPING

Bone Health: Medium–High    Stamina: 2–3    Strength: 2
Flexibility: 2–3

Skipping is a simple but effective aerobic activity that can be used for both recreational and serious endurance training. It has always been much favoured by boxers, as it develops cardio-respiratory endurance and also light evasive footwork. Skipping is an ideal form of home fitness training that can be practised in the garage, on the patio or on any suitable firm surface. All the equipment you need is a skipping rope of the correct length and trainers (or a comfortable pair of well-soled flexible shoes).

Skipping boxer-style is a simple form of skipping on the spot. First of all stand erect, feet together and weight on the toes. The ends of the rope are held in each hand. The main part of the rope is arranged behind the feet for forward skipping, or in front of the feet for backward skipping. In order to swing the rope freely, the arms are held slightly away from the sides and can, if necessary, be raised higher to adjust for the rotation of the rope. As the rope is swung over the head and is about to touch the feet, a hop is made with both feet leaving the floor at the same time. The rope passes under the feet which return to the floor simultaneously. This is high impact exercise. Another and less demanding form of skipping consists of a skip-jump with a rebound. When forward skipping, swing the rope over the head; as it reaches your feet, spring up and down twice on the toes, the first spring being the stronger to clear the rope, the second a small rebound making a 'one-two' rhythm to each swing of the rope. Backward skipping is carried out in similar fashion, with the rope passing under the feet from behind.

Always keep the head and shoulders erect and the feet close together and skip with a relaxed and continuous action. Variations to skipping can be made by skipping over the rope alternating one foot at a time, say for one minute, then skipping with both feet together for another minute. Skipping on one leg only is a demanding plyometric exercise. As you get fitter and your technique improves, increase the exercise time.

STAIR CLIMBING

Bone Health: Medium    Stamina: 2–3    Strength: 2
Flexibility: 1–2

Stair climbing is an energetic, strengthening exercise that is worth considering for an indoor exercise programme. If you can walk quickly or run up a staircase a few times each day, it helps to maintain leg strength and makes you feel good. It is estimated that you use about 15 times more energy to climb stairs, to a set height, than you would use for walking at a similar speed to a distance equal to that height. Going downstairs is, of course, less costly in energy consumption and involves 33 per cent of the energy used to ascend the stairs; but the leg muscles benefit from controlling the descent by working eccentrically (that is, working in a lengthening state).

Climbing stairs is normally a short but quite demanding exercise that could, if continued, make you breathless in a comparatively limited period of time due to the rapid build-up of oxygen debt. The effect on the cardiovascular system and value as an aerobic conditioning exercise can therefore be limited, as it is not normally possible to sustain the exercise period long enough to reap the benefit. However, there are two ways of obtaining a training effect. Firstly, a single flight of stairs can be used if you establish a step cadence that permits the continuous ascent and descent of the stairs, so allowing the exercise to be sustained over a period of time that will ensure aerobic benefits. Secondly, in large buildings, such as high-rise flats where there are many levels, it is feasible to achieve an effective aerobic work-out that could justify a stamina rating of four. You should ensure that the stair inclines are not too severe in step height and angle, and that each landing has a flat area leading to the next ascent to give a less intense phase in the exercise. Even so, such demanding exercises should only be attempted by the very fit.

The principles of overload training can be applied to climbing stairs, by heightened work intensity through increasing the rate or length of your ascent, or by degree of resistance through carrying extra weight such as hand weights or a loaded rucksack.

For those who are attracted to this type of training but do not have access to a flight of steps in their home, there are now various step climbing training machines available in various formats (see page 233). Simple ones are just compact small machines incorporating two low-set pedals attached to two hydraulic cylinders, with variable resistance settings to simulate stepping resistance. At the other end of the range are sturdy, fully framed designs incorporating handlebars for support, hydraulic pedals with non-slip foot pads, perhaps six tension settings, and electronic monitoring with a built-in meter display (showing time, rate, step count, total steps, energy consumption and pulse).

STEP-UPS

Bone Health: Medium–High     Stamina: 2–3     Strength: 2
Flexibility: 1–2

Step-ups are a medium-to-high-impact, demanding form of exercise that develops leg strength and cardio-respiratory endurance. All that is needed is either a sturdy box, bench or firm step about seven inches (18 cm) to 12 inches (30 cm) high The actual height of the step should depend on your height and degree of fitness. First of all, stand erect with head up and arms at the sides facing the step (page 105, exercise 3). Step as follows to the count of four:

| | |
|---|---|
| Count 1 | Place the right foot on the step. |
| Count 2 | As the step-up is made, the left foot is brought up alongside the right and the body straightened. |
| Count 3 | Step down, leading with the right foot. |
| Count 4 | Then step down with the left foot and straighten the body. |

Once you are familiar with the action adopt a good, steady pace so that the movement up and down – on to and from the step – is smooth and rhythmic. It may be possible to complete one repetition every two seconds that will give a target of 30 steps per minute. Change the leading leg every so often so that the workload for each leg is equal. According to your standard of fitness, progressions can be made by:

a. Raising the height of the step slightly, provided the form and rhythm of the movement is not affected.
b. Extending the number of steps taken in each training session.
c. Increasing the cadence of the step-ups (but good form must be retained).

d. Carrying out the exercise with a dumb-bell in each hand or bar-bell held across the shoulders. The weight of each can be gradually increased (but again correct form must always be maintained).

## Step Training

This is a comparatively recent and popular form of low-impact exercise, introduced from the USA, incorporating the use of a low portable step. Though the principle of exercise by stepping on to and down from a raised platform has been around for years, step training is different in that it incorporates a routine of conditioning exercises including stretching exercises. The step can be adjustable, vary in height, perhaps four to six inches, and be made of lightweight polyethylene. Step training is often performed to music but is not too dance orientated. At any one time, one foot always remains in contact with the floor. This puts less stress on joints. Step training can be performed in the comfort of your home, with a video to guide you, or in a class situation.

### HOME CIRCUIT TRAINING

Bone Health: High   Stamina: 3–4   Strength: 3   Flexibility: 3

A basic home circuit should comprise a series of vigorous exercises aiming to exercise the different parts of the body in a set sequence. In addition to developing endurance and strength, the circuit can include exercises that have a high impact value, therefore having a beneficial effect on bone strength. Page 103 explains the principles and methods employed in circuit training.

The basic home circuit shown in figure 44 requires no apparatus apart from a suitable mat, a sturdy box or bench about seven to twelve inches high and a strong chair. It can be used in the garage or on the patio. The six exercises are suitable for beginners. They aim to promote leg, abdominal, arm and shoulder and back strength; and, to a degree, aerobic fitness.

Figure 44: Basic Six-Station Home Exercise Circuit

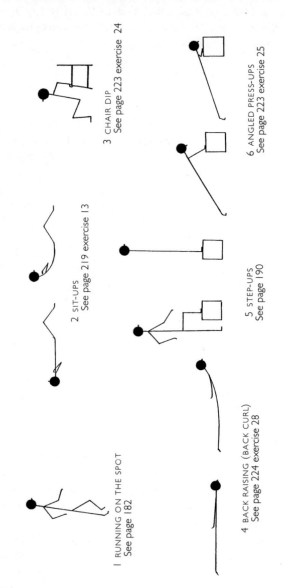

1 RUNNING ON THE SPOT
See page 182

2 SIT-UPS
See page 219 exercise 13

3 CHAIR DIP
See page 223 exercise 24

4 BACK RAISING (BACK CURL)
See page 224 exercise 28

5 STEP-UPS
See page 190

6 ANGLED PRESS-UPS
See page 223 exercise 25

The standard method of testing each individual's fitness at each exercise and establishing their training level is explained at page 104. The programme here is simplified so that after running on the spot for three to five minutes the other five exercises are, according to personal ability, initially performed five to ten times. Do this exercise three or four times a week on alternate days.

Work your way through the following progressions as you feel able, but only move on to the next stage when you are ready to do so. Figure 25 (page 106) shows the type of record card you can maintain.

a. At first, complete the exercise circuit with a pause between each exercise, concentrating on style. Rest, then repeat the circuit to consolidate your technique.
b. Complete one circuit non-stop.
c. Complete two laps of the circuit with a rest between each lap.
d. Complete two laps with no rest between.
e. Complete three laps with a rest between each lap.
f. Complete three laps with no rest between.
g. Further progress can be made by gradually increasing the repetitions for each exercise.

HOME WEIGHT TRAINING

Bone Health: High   Stamina: 2   Strength: 4   Flexibility: 1–2

A home weight-training circuit requires little outlay in cash or equipment. Basically all you need are a set of dumb-bells and a suitable mat. It is possible to buy a family set of dumb-bells to include perhaps three sets of weights, 1.1 kg, 2.3 kg and 4.5 kg. These can be used by the whole family, from young children to teenagers to mum and dad, but note that as adults improve in strength much heavier weights may be required.

Dumb-bells lend themselves to a variety of exercises, particularly those involved with arm and shoulder strength. Start with light dumb-bells that you can handle easily and practise concentrating on the correct technique before

193

commencing training. Once you are completely familiar with the exercise, increase the weight to a load that will permit about 15 repetitions (reps) for that exercise. If you possess a variety of weights at home, progress by exercising gradually and eventually build up to a weight for each exercise that allows you to manage ten to twelve reps. Pages 116–20 outline the principles of weight training, the progressions possible, a beginner's programme and the safety precautions that need to be observed. You can also improvise and use readily available weights such as plastic water bottles, food cans and redundant household containers that have handles, now sand or water filled, all marked according to weight, these afford a variety of dumb-bell-type weights. Even if you do not possess the precise loads that would normally be used to progress, there are useful benefits to be obtained from exercising with improvised weights. For example, such exercises as lateral arm raises or alternate rowing, carried out using cans of baked beans or water bottles, can improve your muscle tone, change your body shape and help to make you slender, firmer and feeling good.

The exercises that follow, figures 45 (opposite) and 46 (page 201), are given as a guide to the simple but effective exercises that can be carried out at home. They include a choice of 11 dumb-bell or improvised hand weight exercises made up of arm and shoulder; trunk; abdominal; back; leg; and lower leg (calf) exercises. These are followed by six exercises using leg weights or resistance.

As with any form of training, always warm up for about five to ten minutes. This period of physical and mental preparation will help you feel ready to start and lessen the risk of accident or injury.

Figure 45: Dumb-bell Exercises

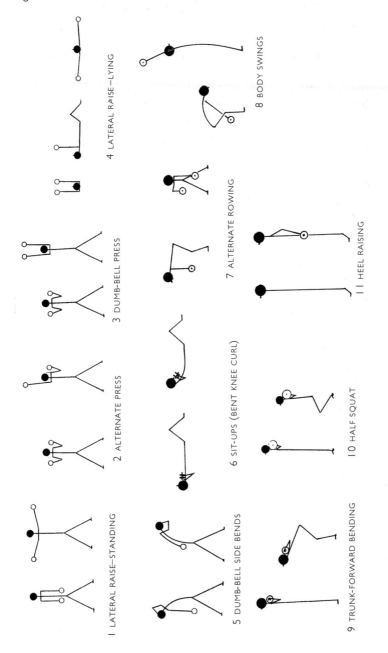

1 LATERAL RAISE—STANDING

2 ALTERNATE PRESS

3 DUMB-BELL PRESS

4 LATERAL RAISE—LYING

5 DUMB-BELL SIDE BENDS

6 SIT-UPS (BENT KNEE CURL)

7 ALTERNATE ROWING

8 BODY SWINGS

9 TRUNK-FORWARD BENDING

10 HALF SQUAT

11 HEEL RAISING

195

## Dumb-bell Exercises

### Arm and Shoulder Exercises

1 Lateral Raise – Standing

*Purpose* To develop shoulder and upper back muscles.
*Starting position* Stand erect with the feet just over shoulder width apart, arms by the sides and a dumb-bell in each hand, palms facing inward.
*Action* Raise the dumb-bells sideways and up with straight arms to shoulder height, at the same time raising the chest high and breathing in as you do so; pause, then lower them under control to the starting position, breathing out at the same time. Repeat.

2 Alternate Press

*Purpose* To develop the shoulders, upper back and muscles at the back of the upper arm.
*Starting position* Stand erect with feet just over shoulder width apart. Or, if necessary to lessen back strain, sit erect. Hold a dumb-bell in each hand, arms bent sideways at shoulder height with the knuckles facing outward.
*Action* Press the right dumb-bell up to arm's length with the knuckles still facing outward, breathing in as you do so. Pause, then lower to the starting position, breathing out at the same time and repeat with the left arm. Continue, alternating the arm action.

3 Dumb-bell Press

*Purpose* To develop the shoulders, upper back and muscles at the back of the upper arm.
*Starting position* Stand erect with the feet just over shoulder width apart or, if necessary, to lessen back strain, sit erect. Hold a dumb-bell in each hand, arms bent sideways at shoulder height with the knuckles facing outward.

*Action* Press the dumb-bells simultaneously up to arm's length with the knuckles still facing outward, lifting the chest high as you do so and breathing in as they are raised. Pause, then lower to the starting position, breathing out at the same time. Repeat.

## 4 Lateral Raise – Lying

*Purpose* To strengthen the chest muscles and front shoulder muscles.
*Starting position* Lie on the back, knees bent and slightly apart, feet on the floor, dumb-bells held at arm's length vertically above each shoulder.
*Action* Lower the dumb-bells together sideways, keeping the arms straight, breathing in as the bells are lowered. Then raise them up to the starting position, breathing out as they are raised. Repeat the exercise.

Note: Initially, comparatively light weights should be used.

## Trunk Exercise

## 5 Dumb-bell Side Bends

*Purpose* To develop muscles at the sides of the trunk and to also make for trunk flexibility.
*Starting position* Stand erect with feet well apart and holding a dumb-bell in the right hand, palm inward, left hand held at the back of the head. Then take up the starting position, with the body bent to the right, but square to the front.
*Action* Breathing in, bend the body strongly to the left but still face the front. Breathe out as the starting position is resumed. After several movements, change the dumb-bell from the right to the left hand and raise the right hand to the back of the head, then repeat the exercise.

## Abdominal Exercise

### 6 Sit-ups (Bent-Knee Curl)

*Purpose* To strengthen and develop the abdominal muscles.
*Starting position* Lie on your back with the feet held or anchored. The knees are bent at about 90°, the feet flat on the floor and a light dumb-bell held high on the chest with both hands.
*Action* Tucking your chin on to your chest, curl as far forward as you can. Breathe out as you sit up, and in as you return to the starting position.

Note: If you are not familiar with sit-ups, practise for some time without the use of any weights and progress slowly.

## Back Exercises

### 7 Alternate Rowing

*Purpose* To develop the muscles of the upper back and arms.
*Starting position* Stand with the feet about shoulder width apart, knees slightly bent to relieve any pressure on the lower back. Holding a dumb-bell in each hand, bend forward from the waist until the trunk is almost parallel with the floor and the dumb-bells, held at arm's length, are directly below each shoulder.
*Action* Raise the right hand to pull the dumb-bell as high as you can, the elbow being parallel with the shoulders. Breathe in as you raise the bell; then lower to the starting position, breathing out as you do so. Repeat with the left hand. Make the action continuous.

### 8 Body Swings

*Purpose* To develop the muscles of the lower back and shoulders.
*Starting position* Stand erect with feet about shoulder width apart and two dumb-bells placed on the floor in front of you. Bend from the knees to pick up the bells, keeping the elbows

and wrists locked in a straight line.

*Action* On the count of 'one' swing the dumb-bells back between the legs. On 'two' swing them in an arc forward and up over the head so that the body is fully extended, but with the elbows and wrists still locked. On 'three' swing the bells in an arc back to position one (between the legs). The movement is continuous and carried out at a moderate cadence.

## 9 Trunk-Forward Bending

*Purpose* To develop the muscles of the lower back, thighs and hips.

*Starting position* Stand with the feet shoulder width apart, one dumb-bell held with both hands behind the neck, or one held at each shoulder.

*Action* Breathing out, bend forward from the hips, keeping the head up and back flat. Allow the knees to bend slightly as the body becomes almost parallel with the floor. Hold for two seconds then, breathing in, return to the starting position and repeat. During the movement, keep the hips forward over the ankles and do not thrust them back so that the weight appears to be on your toes. It is important to commence this exercise with a light weight and then gradually increase the load.

Note: If you have a tendency for back pain *avoid* this exercise.

## Leg Exercise

## 10 Half Squat

*Purpose* To strengthen the thigh and buttock muscles.

*Starting position* Stand with the feet shoulder width apart with a book or wooden block under the heels. A dumb-bell is held in each hand at shoulder level.

*Action* Breathe out as you bend the knees until the thighs are almost parallel to the floor. The back is kept straight. Push up from the lower position by straightening the legs, breathing in as you do so. Repeat.

## Lower Leg (Calf) Exercise

### 11 Heel Raising

*Purpose* To strengthen the calf muscles.
*Starting position* Stand erect.
*Action* Rise up on to the toes, hold, then lower. Progress to standing on one leg, initially with support if required, then again rise on to the toes. Repeat with the other leg. Further progression can be made by the use of weights, perhaps commencing with 2.3 kg weights held in one hand; or at the shoulder, the other hand supporting.

## Exercises with Leg Weights or Against Resistance

Leg weights can be used to strengthen the lower limbs. These weights can take the form of a metal sole strapped to your training shoe, or ankle weights that can be strapped to the ankle. It is possible to improvise and gain the same effect by attaching suitable weights to a mountain boot or similar strong boot.

### 1 Sitting – Knee Extension

*Purpose* To strengthen the thigh (quadriceps) muscles.
*Starting position* Sit upright on the floor, legs straight and trunk either supported by your hands behind you or your back against a wall. A weight is attached to each ankle, a large rolled towel placed under the knees.
*Action* Press the back of the knee of one leg into the towel to fully straighten the leg by contracting the thigh muscles as hard as you can. Hold the tension for two seconds, then relax. Repeat with the other leg.

Figure 46: Exercises with Leg Weights or Against Resistance

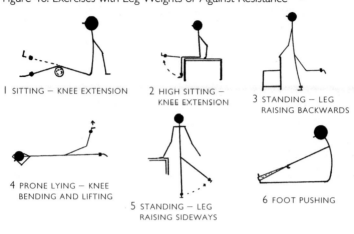

1 SITTING — KNEE EXTENSION

2 HIGH SITTING —
KNEE EXTENSION

3 STANDING — LEG
RAISING BACKWARDS

4 PRONE LYING — KNEE
BENDING AND LIFTING

5 STANDING — LEG
RAISING SIDEWAYS

6 FOOT PUSHING

## 2 High Sitting – Knee Extension

*Purpose* To strengthen the thigh (quadriceps) muscles.
*Starting position* Sit on a high chair or box, feet off the floor, with the knees at 90° and a weight strapped to each ankle.
*Action* Slowly extend one leg until the knee is straight, but keeping the thigh in contact with the seat. Hold the position for about three seconds before slowly lowering the weight back to the starting position. Repeat with the same leg to lift the weight initially about five times, before exercising the other leg.

The number of reps can be gradually increased as can the weight, but take great care not to overload the knee joint. If you experience difficulty in raising the weight, or if the knee cannot be straightened, the weight could be too heavy, putting strain on the joint.

## 3 Standing – Leg Raising Backwards

*Purpose* To strengthen the buttock and hamstring muscles (back of the legs).
*Starting position* Stand erect with a weight on each ankle with support in front, such as a window shelf or sturdy chair.

*Action* Bend one knee to a right angle by pressing the knee backward. Hold, then lower. Alternate the leg movements.

## 4 Prone Lying – Knee Bending and Lifting

*Purpose* To strengthen the buttock and hamstring muscles (back of the legs).
*Starting position* Lie on your front, head on your hands, with weights around each ankle.
*Action* Bend the knees one at a time to a right angle, at the same time lifting the leg upwards from the hip. Alternate the legs.

## 5 Standing – Leg Raising Sideways

*Purpose* To strengthen the muscles of the side of the hip and upper leg.
*Starting position* Stand erect with support to the side, weights on the ankles.
*Action* Keep the body straight and facing forward, body weight on the right leg. Raise the left leg, which stays straight, sideways. Return the leg slowly across the front of the other leg, hold, then raise sideways again before returning to the starting position. Repeat a number of times before changing to the right leg.

## 6 Foot Pushing

*Purpose* To strengthen muscles of the calf.
*Starting position* Sit upright on the floor, legs straight, with back supported if need be. The resistance in this instance is provided by a rubber belt run around the ball of the foot and held in the hands.
*Action* Repeatedly push both feet against the belt. Progress to pushing one foot against the belt, then change to the other foot.

Bone Health: Medium    Stamina: Nil    Strength: 3–4
Flexibility: Nil

The values of isometric exercise have been mentioned previously (see pages 25 and 114) and are now recapped and explained further for the benefit of the home-exerciser.

Isometric exercises can make a useful contribution to a home exercise programme. They are simple to perform, require no equipment and can be carried out virtually anywhere, at any time, in a house or flat. They can be of particular value to the housebound and those suffering from mobility difficulties. People with such problems should first *seek medical advice* before exercising. So should the elderly, or anyone with heart problems or high levels of blood pressure, as isometrics can raise blood pressure during the actual exercise.

Isometrics aim to develop muscle strength and tone by exercising muscles against an immovable load. The concept is based on the fact that a six-second maximum contraction against a static force will bring about the recruitment of the maximum number of muscle fibres possible in a muscle, but only in that one fixed position. Being static, isometrics do not contribute to the development of endurance or flexibility. However, they can serve as a useful break in the day's routine or as part of your indoor exercise programme – perhaps with conditioning exercises to give mobility; and stationary cycling or running to maintain aerobic fitness, resulting in a balanced cross training programme.

Note that it is important to build up isometric tension *gradually*.

## Method and Progression

The effectiveness of an isometric exercise programme depends on the length of time, counted in seconds, that the muscles are contracted (up to five or six); the degree of vigour of the contractions; and the frequency with which the programme is carried out. Like all types of exercise, progressions should be gradual.

Initially, the tension applied to each exercise should be held for about a second – the time it takes you to say 'one and two' – and be performed below maximum exertion. Eventually it can be built up to six seconds, with tension held at maximum exertion. It is believed that attempting to hold the tension beyond that length of time would have little benefit, for it is not possible to maintain the involvement of the maximum number of muscle fibres. Research to date into the most effective training methods has shown that five to ten contractions at maximal strength, held for five seconds, with a training frequency of three days a week, registers some of the best improvements.

As with all exercise, first of all make sure that you are performing the exercise correctly. This is particularly important with isometrics, as their effect can be easily lost if bad technique is applied. If need be, check your positions in a mirror. Isometric exercises require that certain muscles or muscle groups are isolated, so initially they may feel a little strange to perform until the body's nervous system becomes familiar with the muscle action involved. Once learnt and practised, however, the benefits will soon become apparent. An isometric programme should be based on exercises that benefit the different parts of the body:

> Neck
> Arm and shoulder
> Fingers and wrist
> Trunk
> Leg

Although the following exercises (see page 206, figure 47) are suitable for inclusion in your home exercise programme, some of them can be done inconspicuously at other times when you have a few minutes to spare – perhaps during working hours, waiting for a bus or train, or travelling in a car or aeroplane. You will find they make you feel good.

## Neck Exercises

### 1 Side Neck

Sit or stand upright, facing forward, with the head erect. Raise your right arm and place the base of the right palm against the head, just above the right ear. Push the head towards the right, but resist with the palm so that no appreciable movement takes place. Hold the exercise for the count of 'one and two'. Repeat the exercise on the left side using the left palm.

### 2 Front Neck

Sit or stand upright, facing forward, with the head held erect. Raise the arms up to place the palms of your hands on the right and left sides of the forehead, fingers uppermost, the hands just touching. Push the head forward, but resist with the palms so that no appreciable movement takes place. Hold the exercise for the count of 'one and two'.

### 3 Back neck

Sit or stand upright, facing forward, with the head held erect. Raise both arms to place both palms across the back of the head, fingers intertwined. Push the head backwards, but resist with the strongly intertwined fingers so that no appreciable movement takes place. Hold the exercise for the count of 'one and two'.

## Arm and Shoulder Exercises

### 4 Arm Pushing

Sit or stand upright. Raise the elbows up to shoulder height and place the left fist, knuckles facing upward, just in front of the chest and against the cupped palm of the right hand. Keeping the elbows at shoulder height, push the left fist

Figure 47: Isometric Programme

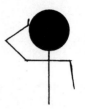

1 SIDE NECK

2 FRONT NECK

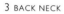

3 BACK NECK

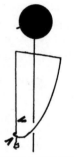

7 SINGLE ARM RAISE

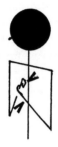

8 SINGLE ARM
EXTENSION

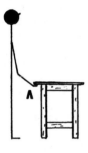

9 ELBOW FLEXION

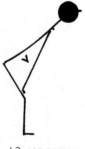

12 ABDOMINAL

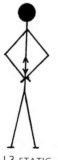

13 STATIC
ABDOMINAL

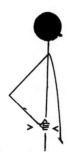

14 LATERAL TENSION

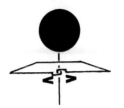

4 ARM PUSHING

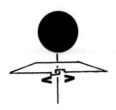

5 ARM PULLS

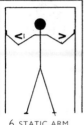

6 STATIC ARM EXTENSION

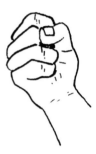

10 FINGER SQUEEZE

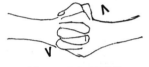

11 WRIST TWISTING

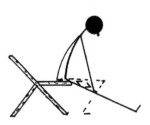

15 STATIC QUADRICEPS

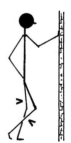

16 HIP AND THIGH EXERCISE

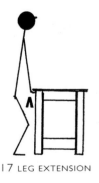

17 LEG EXTENSION

against the palm of the right hand so that there is no appreciable movement. Hold the exercise for the count of 'one and two'.

## 5 Arm Pulls

Sit or stand upright. Raise the elbows to shoulder height, then fold the fingers of each hand and interlock them just in front of the chest, knuckles facing the opposite direction. Pull with both arms against the interlocked fingers that resist all movement, but making sure the elbows remain at shoulder height. Hold the exercise for the count of 'one and two'.

## 6 Static Arm Extension

Stand in a *wide* door frame or doorway where you can, with comfort, raise your arms to place the palms of the hands at shoulder height with arms bent, on the door frame or walls. Push outward against the door frame or walls. Hold the exercise for the count of 'one and two'.

## 7 Single-Arm Raise

Stand upright, arms by the sides, right fist clenched. Move the left arm across to grip the right wrist with the left hand. Keeping the right arm straight, try to raise the right arm forward and up, but resist with the left arm so that there is no appreciable movement. Hold the exercise for the count of 'one and two'. Repeat the exercise, this time with the left wrist grasped.

## 8 Single-Arm Extension

Sit or stand upright. Clench the right fist, then bend the right arm and hold it with the palm facing the chest in front of the right side, with the elbow tucked against the upper body. Grasp the right wrist with the left hand, left elbow held firmly against the left side of the chest. The knuckles of the left hand face forward. Push with the right arm in a forward and downward direction, but resist with the left hand so that no appreciable movement takes place. Hold the exercise for the count of 'one and two'. Repeat the exercise, this time with the left wrist grasped.

### 9 Elbow Flexion

Stand upright, facing an immovable bench top or desk, and grasp the underside firmly with your hands shoulder width apart. Try to 'lift' the structure by flexing the arms only. Hold the exercise for the count of 'one and two'.

### Fingers and Wrist Exercises

### 10 Finger Squeeze

Sit, stand or lie holding a squash ball or a large India rubber in one or both hands. Squeeze the squash ball(s) or rubber(s) as hard as you can, one hand at a time. Hold the exercise for the count of 'one and two'.

### 11 Wrist Twisting

Sit or stand. Place the palms of your hands together with the fingers forward and resting lightly on your tummy. Firmly intertwine the fingers, knuckles facing forward. Twist the left hand and wrist towards you, resisting by twisting the right hand and wrist away. Hold the exercise for the count of 'one and two'. Repeat the exercise in the opposite direction.

## Trunk Exercises

### 12 Abdominal

Stand erect, feet just a little way apart, knees slightly bent. Bend forward from the hips to place the heel of each hand on each thigh with fingers inward, just above the kneecaps. Hollow the back slightly. Try to bend further at the hips, drawing in the tummy muscles as you simultaneously resist with the hands pressing against the thighs so that there is no appreciable movement. Hold the exercise for the count of 'one and two'.

### 13 Static Abdominal

Begin by lying on your back, sitting or standing, hands just above the hips so as to feel the tension exerted on the muscles. Tighten the tummy as hard as you can Hold the exercise for the usual count of 'one and two'. The exercise will help to give muscle tone and also an ongoing awareness of your increasing or decreasing waist size!

### 14 Lateral Tension

Stand erect, feet just apart. Place the right palm, fingers facing forward, on the top of the pelvic bone. Push the palm against the hip, but resisting with the hip so that no appreciable movement takes place. Hold the exercise for the count of 'one and two'. Repeat the exercise with the left palm on the left hip.

## Leg Exercises

### 15 Static Quadriceps

This exercise can be done lying, sitting or standing and is designed to strengthen the big muscles in the front of the thigh.

If you are sitting on a chair, sit on the edge of the chair and extend your right leg so that it is straight and supported by the heel with the muscles relaxed. Now tense the big thigh muscles of the right leg as hard as you can, the kneecap being drawn back. The degree of tension applied can be felt if your right hand grips the muscles lightly just above the knee. Hold the exercise for the count of 'one and two'. Repeat the exercise with the left leg.

## 16 Hip and Thigh Exercise

Stand erect about two feet from your support (perhaps a wall or chair). Place the left hand on the support to assist balance. Take the body weight on the right leg and bend the right knee slightly with the right foot flat on the floor. Cross the left leg over the right so that the calf of the left leg is against the right shin, with the toes of the left foot touching the floor. Push forward with right thigh, but press back with the left leg so that no appreciable movement is made. Hold the position for the count of 'one and two'. Repeat the exercise with the left leg taking the body weight. Once your balance is established you may not need support.

## 17 Leg Extension

Stand with feet apart, knees slightly flexed, facing a fairly low work bench or counter top that is immovable. Grasp the underside with your hands shoulder width apart and arms straight. Try to 'lift' the structure, but keep the arms and back straight and only use your legs. Hold the exercise for the count of 'one and two'.

## CONDITIONING EXERCISES (CALLISTHENICS)

Bone Health: Medium–High     Stamina: 2–3     Strength: 2–3
Flexibility: 3–4

Conditioning exercises, or callisthenics, are set exercises that aim to improve body strength, flexibility and co-ordination. If they are carried out continuously with sufficient vigour to raise the heart rate – but not so as to reach a state of breathlessness – and continued for more than 15 minutes, aerobic benefits can be derived. Conditioning exercises are ideal for indoor training, requiring little or no equipment other than a mat or chair, and can be performed in a comparatively small space. Progressive callisthenics are exercises where the degree of difficulty is gradually increased as the fitness and ability of the individual improves.

## Grades

The exercises that follow (see page 216, figure 48) are graded to give three progressive levels. Level one is suitable for fit beginners; in level three the intensity of effort required is much greater. Note that the exercise programme outlined is *not suitable* for the infirm or elderly.

The programme is made up of eight exercise categories, planned in a set order and intended to exercise and benefit the various parts of the body. In some category levels a choice of exercise is given. The order is significant, as it ensures a balanced training session allowing the part of the body just exercised to recover while the next exercise, affecting a different part of the body, is being attempted.

The exercise categories are carried out in the following sequence:

| CATEGORY NUMBER | EXERCISE CATEGORY |
| --- | --- |
| 1 | Arm and Shoulder Mobility |
| 2 | Leg Strength (Medium to High Impact) |
| 3 | Trunk Flexibility – Lateral Movements |
| 4 | Abdominal Strength |
| 5 | Trunk Flexibility – Horizontal Movements |
| 6 | Leg Strength and Mobility |
| 7 | Shoulder and Upper Arm Strength |
| 8 | Back Strength |

## High Impact Exercises

It is believed that *any* exercise undertaken by persons who have lived a mainly sedentary lifestyle, particularly women, will have some positive effect on bone mass and health. However, the inclusion of high impact exercises in a home exercise programme, being weight-bearing, can play a direct role in promoting bone health. The inclusion of specific medium to high impact leg-strengthening exercises (as in exercise category two), which are dynamic, should have benefits for the development and maintenance of bone health. These benefits relate not only to the leg and hip bones, but to the general skeletal system.[1] Many of the other exercises listed in this home exercise programme have been selected to gain the benefits from dynamic controlled movement relating to bone health.

## Method and Progression

The programme should be preceded by a warm-up and followed by a gentle warm-down (see pages 57–8). There are three or more exercises included under each of the eight categories. Commence with the exercise given at level one in each category. As the fitness standard of home exercise participants can vary greatly, and so can the age of those involved, exercises are practised initially by carrying out five to ten repetitions aiming for good form and rhythm.

Your aim at each exercise should be to do the exercise correctly without undue strain. The movements should be controlled, not forced. If during the exercise you feel unduly breathless, *stop exercising*. If need be, have a short break between exercises. A little discomfort may be experienced at first as you gently exercise unaccustomed muscles and tendons, but if you experience pain in joints or tendons, stop and *avoid* that exercise. Following several sessions of initial practice you may wish, according to your personal fitness level and ability, to adjust the number of repetitions for each

---

[1] Those who are overweight, or suffer from joint problems where the cartilage may have commenced to wear, should avoid high impact exercises and switch to those that have a low impact effect.

exercise. This can be done by adding between two and five repetitions at the end of each week, or when you are ready.

Eventually you will feel able to move up to the next exercise level. After progressing from the initial level, practise with five to ten repetitions at the new level, then increase the repetitions as before and record your progress (see page 226, figure 49). Those seeking to get the maximum training effect from their indoor conditioning programme should apply the following principles:

   a. Increase the number of reps for each exercise.
   b. Reduce any resting time between exercises, eventually achieving a continuous, vigorous but controlled session so that one exercise flows into the other.
   c. Repeat the series of exercises a second time after a short rest.
   d. Repeat the series with no rest.

## Category 1: Arm and Shoulder Mobility

### 1 Arm Circling Level 1

Stand erect with the feet shoulder width apart. Raise the arms up in front, then back close to the ears and down so that the hands brush the thighs to complete a large circle. Make the movement smooth and rhythmical, starting with five to ten circles forwards and backwards.

### 2 Angled Arm Swings Level 2

Stand with the feet shoulder width apart, arms by the sides. Raise both arms up in front to shoulder height, fists lightly clenched, knuckles facing outwards. Now swing both arms sideways and backwards as far as you comfortably can, but do *not* make any jerking or ballistic movements. The hands should be a little higher than the shoulders at the end of the movement. Swing the arms back to the forward position, then down to the sides. Now repeat the exercise to the rhythmic count of four. Perform the exercise five to ten times to start with.

### 3 Elbow Circling *Level 3*

Stand erect with the feet shoulder width apart. Place your fingers on each shoulder. Rotate both elbows backwards so that the elbows describe as wide a circle as possible. Repeat the same movement forwards. Making the movements smooth and rhythmical, start with five to ten circles each way.

### 4 Backward Reaching *Level 3*

Stand erect with feet astride, arms by the sides. Simultaneously raise the right arm up then back and the left arm down and back, pressing as far back as is comfortable. Hold to the count of 'one and two' and then swing to reverse the arms with the same count. Keep the back straight and the movement rhythmical, starting with six to ten movements (three to five to each side).

## Category 2: Leg Strength (Medium to High Impact)

### 5 Stride Jumping *Level 1*

Stand erect, feet together, arms by the sides. Spring lightly to land on the toes, with the feet astride, and simultaneously swing both arms up sideways to clap hands above your head. Rebound to the starting position. Perform five to ten times to start with.

### 6 Stride Jumping with Arm Swings *Level 2*

Stand erect, feet together, arms by the sides. Spring lightly to land on the toes with the feet astride, arms simultaneously raised sideways just above shoulder height. Rebound back to the starting position. Then keep bouncing but alternating the arm action with arm swings forward to shoulder height, then back (to make one count). Perform the exercise five to ten times to start with.

Figure 48: Conditioning Exercise Programme

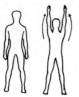 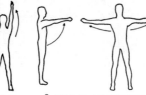  

1 ARM CIRCLING    2 ANGLED ARM SWINGS    3 ELBOW CIRCLING    4 BACKWARD REACHING

 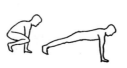

7 SQUAT JUMPS    8 SQUAT THRUSTS    9 BURPEES

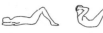 

14 SIT-UPS WITH HANDS BESIDE THE HEAD    15 SIT-UPS WITH ARMS STRETCHED    16 TRUNK ROTATION WITH RIGHT-ANGLE ARM SWINGS

21 HALF SQUATS    22 ARM FLEXION AND EXTENSION    23 ANGLED PRESS-UPS

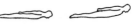

28 BACK RAISING (BACK CURL)

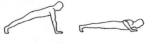

27 PRESS-UPS

29 BACK RAISING (BACK CURL) WITH HANDS BEHIND HEAD

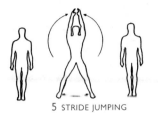

5 STRIDE JUMPING

6 STRIDE JUMPING WITH ARM SWINGS

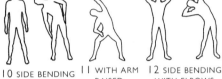

10 SIDE BENDING

11 WITH ARM RAISED

12 SIDE BENDING WITH ELBOWS RAISED

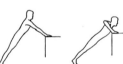

13 SIT-UPS WITH ARMS ON CHEST

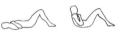

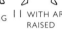

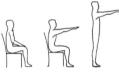

17 TRUNK ROTATION WITH ELBOWS UP

18 TRUNK ROTATION WITH ELBOWS HIGH

19 SKI-PUSH

20 CHAIR SQUAT

24 BASIC CHAIR DIPS

25 MODIFIED ANGLED PRESS-UPS

26 ADVANCED CHAIR DIPS

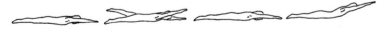

30 BACK, LEG AND ARM RAISING

31 BACK RAISING (BACK CURL) WITH ARMS EXTENDED

### 7 Squat Jumps *Level 3*

Stand erect, feet slightly apart. Keeping your back straight, bend the knees to no more than 90°. Then leap vertically as high as you can with arms extended upwards. Land lightly into the squat position and rebound into the next leap. Perform the exercise five times to start with.

### 8 Squat Thrusts *Level 3*

Assume a squatting position, hands flat on the floor, head up. Thrust the legs back to the press-up position, legs and body straight. Then, with a rebound, bring both legs forward so that the knees touch the elbows. Repeat the movement at a steady pace for five to ten reps. This is an exercise for the younger and more agile.

### 9 Burpees *Level 3*

Stand with the feet together, arms by the sides, head up. Exercise to the count of one to four. On 'one' squat down, palms flat on the floor about shoulder width apart. On 'two' thrust the legs backward with a hop to assume the raised press-up position. On 'three' return with a hop to the squat position. On 'four' return to the starting position. The exercise should be carried out at a moderate speed and initially performed with five to ten repetitions. It is a demanding exercise (best avoided by older people) that, in addition to strengthening legs and hips, can contribute to cardio-respiratory fitness.

### Category 3: Trunk Flexibility – Lateral Movements

### 10 Side Bending *Level 1*

Stand erect with the feet shoulder width apart, toes pointing forward and hands by the sides. Bend gently to the right, so that the right hand follows the line of an imaginary trouser seam down the outside of the leg as far as it can. Do not lean forwards or backwards. Return to the starting position and repeat to the left. Repeat five to ten times each side.

*Note: If you have a tendency for back trouble do not progress to exercises 11 and 12 below but continue with this exercise.*

### 11 Side Bending with Arm Raised *Level 2*

Stand erect, feet wide apart and knees slightly bent. Place the right hand on the right thigh and raise the left arm over the head. Now lift and gently bend from the waist to the right. Hold briefly, then return to vertical, change arms and bend to the left. Repeat five to ten times each side.

### 12 Side Bending with Elbows Raised *Level 3*

Stand erect with the feet about shoulder width apart, toes pointing slightly outward and elbows raised with hands clasped together at the back of head. Bend gently sideways to the right as far as you can go. Do not lean forwards or backwards. Return to the starting position, then repeat to the left. Repeat initially five to ten times each side.

Note: This exercise should *only* be attempted by the fit and supple, and with *no* bouncing or jerking movements.

### Category 4: Abdominal Strength

### 13 Sit-ups with Arms on Chest *Level 1*

Lie on your back with your feet supported, knees at about 90°. The hands are placed across the chest. Breathing out, raise your head and shoulders off the floor and slowly curl up towards the knees. Hold the position briefly, then slowly return to the starting position, breathing in as you do so. Initially repeat the exercise five to ten times.

### 14 Sit-ups with Hands Beside the Head *Level 2*

Lie on your back with your feet supported, knees about 90°
and slightly apart. The hands are placed at the sides of the
head above the ears. Breathing out, tuck your chin into your
chest. Slowly raise the head, then shoulders, off the floor until
the elbows are close to the knees. Hold the position briefly,
then slowly return to the starting position, breathing in as you
do so. Initially repeat the exercise five to 10 times.

### 15 Sit-ups with Arms Stretched *Level 3*

Lie on your back with the feet supported, knees at about 90°
and slightly apart, arms stretched out on the floor behind your
head. Breathing out, slowly curl the head and shoulders. Bring
the arms up and over the head to reach the floor between the
feet, then slowly return to the starting position, breathing in
as you do so. Do not jerk the arms over the head. Initially
repeat the exercise five to ten times.

### Category 5: Trunk Flexibility – Horizontal Movements

### 16 Trunk Rotation with Right-Angle Arm Swings *Level 1*

Stand erect with the feet about shoulder width apart, toes
pointing forward, arms by the side. On the count of 'one', gently swing the right arm – with the fist clenched, thumb uppermost – forward to shoulder height. Keeping the hips facing forwards, continue the gentle swing now to the right, slightly
higher than shoulder level, simultaneously twisting the trunk
and turning the head to the right so that the body rotates
('two'). Swing the arm back and rotate the trunk to face the
front ('three'), then lower arms to the starting position ('four').
Repeat to the left. Now make the movements smooth and
rhythmic. There should be *no* jerking force or ballistic movement at the end of the arm swing. Initially repeat the movement five to ten times to each side.

### 17 Trunk Rotation with Elbows Up *Level 2*

Stand erect, feet about shoulder width apart, elbows at shoulder height in front with hands clasped. Gently twist to the right as far as you comfortably can, keeping the knees locked. Return to face the front, then twist to the left. There should be *no* jerking or ballistic movement at the end of each twist. Initially repeat the movement five times to each side.

### 18 Trunk Rotation with Elbows High *Level 3*

Stand erect, feet about shoulder width apart, hands clasped at the back of the head, and elbows back. Gently twist to the right as far as you can go with comfort, keeping the knees locked to make a firm base. Return to face the front, then twist to the left. There should be *no* jerking or ballistic movement at the end of each twist. Initially make five movements to each side.

### Category 6: Leg Strength and Mobility

### 19 Ski-push *Level 1*

Stand erect, feet hip width apart, toes pointing forward. Raise the arms out in front to head height. Now pull the arms back and down in a semi-circular movement, bending the hips and knees at the same time as if you were propelling yourself on cross-country skis – the arms finishing straight out behind you. Swing the arms back up to the start of the ski movement, straightening the body as you do so. As with actual skiing, the movement should be smooth and rhythmic. Initially perform the exercise five to ten times.

### 20 Chair Squat *Level 2*

Sit upright on a chair or box about 20 inches high, with your feet comfortably apart, flat on the floor with the toes pointing slightly outward, and your hands resting on your thighs.

Keeping the head up and back straight, slowly stand up from the chair. As you do so, raise the arms out in front and keep them there. Now lower yourself onto the chair, reversing the process. Initially do the exercise five to ten times. To make the exercise slightly more difficult, fold your arms across your chest.

### 21 Half Squats Level 3

Stand with your feet just wider than hip width apart, toes pointing slightly outward. Now raise the arms in front. Keeping your back straight, head up and feet flat on the floor, bend the knees so that you sink to a squatting position with the thighs almost parallel to the floor. Return to the starting position and repeat. Initially perform the exercise five to ten times. The exercise can be varied by placing the hands lightly on the back of the head or crossed in front of the chest; or, to make it harder, by carrying a weight.

### Category 7: Shoulder and Upper Arm Strength

### 22 Arm Flexion and Extension Level 1

Stand erect with the feet shoulder width apart, arms by the sides. On the count of 'one' raise the arms to tense them dynamically in a tight half-bent position at the shoulders with fists clenched. Initially hold the position for two seconds, then stretch the arms out away from the sides with fingers stretched at just above shoulder height for two seconds ('two') before returning to the half-bent position for two seconds ('three'), then back to the starting position ('four'). Initially perform the exercise five to ten times.

This can be adapted as an isometric exercise. The tension exerted in the arm-bent position should be just below maximum, then initially held for one second, building up to five seconds – but repeated no more than five times.

This exercise can also be developed into a rhythmic combination with exercise 10 (Side Bending) where the arm flexion and extension is performed to the count of 'four', then followed by side bending to the same count. In this instance there is little isometric effect.

### 23 Angled Press-ups *Level 2*

With arms extended at shoulder width apart, stand several feet from a wall. Lean against the wall, hands still at shoulder width, fingers pointing up. The body is kept straight. Now bend the arms until the forehead almost touches the wall, then straighten to raise the body back to the starting position. The difficulty can be increased by moving the feet back, so altering the angle of the body. Initially perform the exercise five to ten times.

### 24 Basic Chair Dips *Level 2*

This exercise will strengthen the muscles at the back of the arms (triceps). Use a sturdy chair or a bench of similar height. Sit on the edge of the chair or bench, hands gripping the edge, knuckles facing forward. Now move your torso forward so that your bottom comes off the chair, feet flat on the floor and weight on the hands. Lower your bottom towards the floor by bending the arms to 90° (but not to touch the floor), then straighten the arms to raise the body. Repeat the exercise five to ten times to start with.

### 25 Modified Angled Press-up *Level 2–3*

Grip the edge of a bench, window sill or sturdy wide-based chair, with your arms shoulder width apart. Move the feet backwards until the body is straight and angled at about 45°, being supported by the toes and arms which are kept straight. Now lower the chest and almost touch the support by bending the arms. Raise the body back to the starting position by straightening the arms. Initially perform the exercise five to ten times. The degree of difficulty can be increased by using a lower support.

## 26 Advanced Chair Dips *Level 3*

With your back towards a sturdy chair, grip the edge, with your knuckles facing forward. The heels are on the floor, legs straight, arms bent to about 90° and your weight is on your hands. Raise the body by strengthening the arms, then lower. Repeat the exercise five to ten times to start with.

## 27 Press-ups *Level 3*

The body is supported by the toes and the hands which are positioned under the shoulders, fingers facing forward with the arms, body and legs straight. Keeping the legs and body straight, bend the elbows until the chest almost touches the floor, then straighten the arms to raise the body back to its starting position. The degree of difficulty can be increased by raising the feet on to a low box, bench or chair. Initially perform the exercise five to ten times.

## Category 8: Back Strength

*In the following exercises, breathe out as you raise the upper body off the floor; then in, as you slowly lower the body. Do not attempt these exercises if you suffer from back pain or back problems.*

## 28 Back Raising (Back Curl) *Level 1*

Lie on your front face down, with your hands clasped behind your back, feet just apart and supported. Keeping the chin into the chest, raise your head and shoulders off the floor, hold the position for three seconds, then lower back to the starting position. Initially perform the exercise five to ten times.

29 Back Raising (Back Curl) with Hands Behind Head *Level 2*

Lie on your front face down, with your hands clasped behind the head, feet just apart and supported. Keeping the chin into the chest, raise your head and shoulders up off the floor, keeping the hands clasped behind the head. Hold the position for three seconds, then lower back to the starting position. Initially perform the exercise five to ten times.

30 Back, Leg and Arm Raising *Level 2*

Lie face down, arms stretched over the head, fingers pointed. Raise your right arm and left leg as far as you can with comfort, breathing out as you do so. Hold for two seconds, then breathe in as you slowly lower the arm and leg to the floor. Repeat, using the left arm and right leg to count as one movement. Perform the exercise four to ten times to start with.

31 Back Raising (Back Curl) with Arms Extended *Level 3*

Lie face down with the arms fully extended out in front of you, feet just apart and supported. Keeping the chin in, lift the arms, head and shoulders off the floor. Hold the position for three seconds, then gently lower to the starting position. Initially perform the exercise five to ten times.

Figure 49: Conditioning Exercise Record Card

| EXERCISE CAT.NO. | EXERCISE CATEGORY | LEVEL | EXERCISE | EXERCISE DAYS/REPS | | | | | | | | | | | | |
|---|---|---|---|---|---|---|---|---|---|---|---|---|---|---|---|---|
| | | | | 1 | 2 | 3 | 4 | 5 | 6 | 7 | 8 | 9 | 10 | 11-12 | 13 | 14 |
| 1 | Arm and Shoulder Mobility | 1 | Arm Circling | 5 | 5 | 5 | 8 | 8 | 8 | | | | | | | |
| 2 | Leg Strength | 1 | Stride Jumping | 8 | 8 | 8 | 10 | 10 | 10 | | | | | | | |
| 3 | Trunk Flexibility (Lateral) | 1 | Side Bending | 5 | 5 | 5 | 8 | 8 | 8 | | | | | | | |
| 4 | Abdominal Strength | 1 | Sit-ups, Arms on Chest | 5 | 5 | 5 | 7 | 7 | 7 | | | | | | | |
| 5 | Trunk Flexibility (Horizontal) | 1 | Trunk Rotation with Right-Angle Arm Swings | 5 | 5 | 5 | 8 | 8 | 8 | | | | | | | |
| 6 | Leg Strength and Mobility | 1 | Ski-push | 8 | 8 | 8 | 11 | 11 | 11 | | | | | | | |
| 7 | Shoulder and Upper Arm | 1 | Arm Flexion and Extension | 6 | 6 | 6 | 9 | 9 | 9 | | | | | | | |
| 8 | Back Strength | 1 | Back Raising | 5 | 5 | 5 | 7 | 7 | 7 | | | | | | | |

Bone Health: Medium–High     Stamina: 2–3     Strength: 1–2
Flexibility: 3–4

Aerobic dancing is performed to the stimulating rhythm of disco music that, by its powerful pulse, motivates effort and helps the performer to 'keep going'. The concept of exercise to music is far from new, for the value of body movement stimulated by rhythm has long been realised. In the days when sailors lived below decks in cramped, damp conditions, encouragement was given for the crew to exercise regularly and vigorously on deck in the fresh air. This helped them maintain bodily strength and endurance in order to operate the sails and rigging effectively, often in adverse conditions. It is on record that Captain Bligh of the *Bounty*, on his epic voyage to the South Seas in 1787, took with him a semi-blind fiddler to provide music for these exercise sessions. Claims have recently been made that perhaps Captain Bligh was responsible for the origin of the aerobic dance!

The exercises in aerobic dancing are normally of a moderate intensity, but strung together in dance form and repeated many times. The result is continuous movement that provides an excellent and enjoyable form of aerobic training which also has beneficial effects on body shape and flexibility. Participants feel fitter, become trimmer and get firmer. Aerobic classes are very popular with women. Multi-level sessions are run at many sports centres for all abilities and ages. If you do decide to attend, you may need to try a few classes to discover the one that suits you. The most common problems are the music being too fast or too loud; and the mixture of varying fitness levels of individuals in the group, so that only a few really benefit from the session. Some classes are divided into high and low impact.

You do not need to join a centre or club to do aerobics. Video tapes are readily available at most major stores. But first of all you should obtain the advice of a fully qualified instructor, so that the tape you purchase is suitable for your ability level and there is no possibility of you attempting exercises that could prove too difficult or have harmful effects.

Aerobic sessions are also broadcast on television.

A well-planned aerobic exercise session will contain a suitable warm-up phase; then a fairly intense activity period that should raise the heart rate for some 20 minutes or more and aim to develop cardio-respiratory fitness; followed by exercises that aim to develop strength and all-round body flexibility. The sessions should conclude with a warming-down phase, including gentle stretching. Those people new to aerobic dance exercises who are overweight or are of mature years will require a very gentle introduction. The exercises performed should place minimal stress on joints and have little risk of injury. Hopping and skipping movements are not suitable for these categories of home-exerciser. The exercises practised must be of the low impact type, where one foot is always kept in contact with the floor. Even though low impact aerobics are not high intensity exercises, if performed for a sustained period of time – say 45 minutes to an hour – and repeated regularly, they can have beneficial effects on cardio-respiratory fitness.

It is believed that an increase in physical effort made by women who have led a sedentary lifestyle can improve their bone health. Low impact aerobics can make a contribution in this area. High impact aerobics involve more dynamic body movements including the action of jumping, hopping and skipping. They also entail controlled but forceful landings. For those who are fit, strong and so able to tolerate such bone-stressing activity, there are well-defined benefits to be gained from these exercises.

## INDOOR TRAINING: A SIMPLE GUIDE TO EXERCISE TRAINING MACHINES

The qualities of strength, stamina and speed can, as explained in this book, be developed and maintained with the use of little or no equipment. For example, where strength is sought, the use of body weight or improvised weights or resistance can help achieve the aim. Nevertheless there are many who would like to use or purchase some form of exercise machine related to the aspects of fitness they are seeking, perhaps to use at the local sports centres or practise with at home. The area of

Figure 50: Exercise Training Equipment

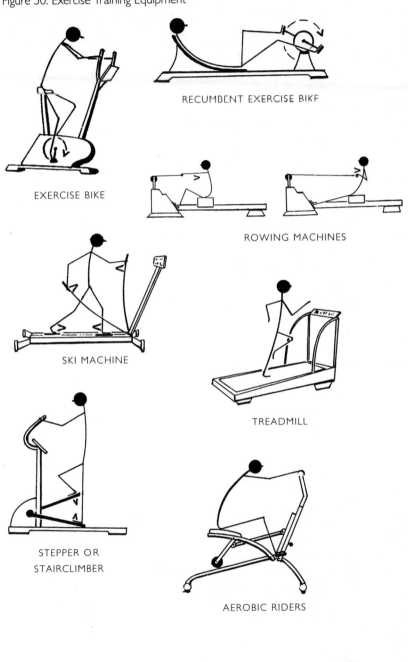

RECUMBENT EXERCISE BIKE

EXERCISE BIKE

ROWING MACHINES

SKI MACHINE

TREADMILL

STEPPER OR
STAIRCLIMBER

AEROBIC RIDERS

exercise training machines is an expanding industry and the types and designs are ever increasing, as is scientific research related to fitness training.

As many people exercise to lose weight, it is useful when using training machines to know your body weight in kilograms, even if you think in imperial scales. Some more sophisticated aerobic training machines, incorporating electronic monitors, require the exerciser to programme his/her weight in kilograms when starting to exercise, so enabling the machine to calculate how many calories can be consumed in each training session. One of the problems with indoor training, particularly when using training machines, is the possibility of boredom. Hence the value of cross-training programmes (see pages 180 and 246). Where available, the use of several types of training machines or switching to different indoor exercises can help keep the mind stimulated, so avoiding boredom, and also exercise different muscle groups.

The details of exercise training machines described here are intended to give the reader a brief guide to the attributes of each form of training, including the beneficial effects related to the respective components of fitness. As with all forms of training, safety should *never* be overlooked (see pages 115 and 236).

## Exercise Bikes

Of all the training machines available in a gym perhaps the first to use should be the stationary cycle, as it is easier to cycle than run, row or step. It is a form of low impact exercise that, when commenced at a steady speed, can contribute to the warm-up – ensuring the blood is flowing freely around the body, the heart rate is gradually increased and body temperature raised. Stationary cycling can be easily adapted to meet a wide range of fitness levels.

Stationary cycles increase aerobic fitness and tone up muscles in the hips, thighs, buttocks and legs. They are avaiable as relatively simple machines or those that have highly informative electronic monitors. They can vary in design to incorporate adjustable friction belt, magnetic or fan resistance and chain or belt drive with fully enclosed mechanisms for added safety. Some are dual or triple action that also make for upper body exercise. Design features should include an adjustable saddle and handlebars and adjustable resistance, pedal straps, speedometer and distance meter. More expensive models will have electronic consoles to include timer, calorie burn and ear sensor pulse monitor. Easy grip controls can allow the rider to adjust resistance accurately through perhaps eight resistance settings. Some even include different pre-set motivational programmes and automatic variation of pedalling intensity.

Recumbent exercise cycles are another form of static cycle, but where the rider adopts an almost prone position. The legs are elevated slightly and support is given to the back, so eliminating pressure points on the back and buttocks. The machine can be suited for those with back trouble (under medical direction) and the older exerciser. Like racing and street recumbent cycles, much body power can be transmitted to the pedals. Recumbent cycle features can include enclosed belt drive and magnetic resistance with comfortable, smooth, quiet pedalling.

When commencing cycling, set the resistance to make for comfortable cycling. A high rate of resistance will demand hard, fast pedalling to attain a target speed (see pages 185–7).

## Rowing Machines

Rowing machines offer a uniquely effective form of low to medium impact exercise that will improve aerobic fitness and also strengthen most muscle groups: abdomen, back, arms and legs. Modern designs incorporate pivoting footplates; easily adjusted hydraulic or air resistance; simulated double individual oars or a cable-attached hand bar; and a smooth, silent, sliding seat on runners. Additional features can include an electronic console to monitor time, strokes per minute, calorie-burn and distance. Some machines even give an audible stroke. More advanced designs suitable for the athlete may incorporate a heavy-flywheel, silent magnetic brake to ensure a smooth stroke and the feel of natural rowing. An electronic meter may give the extra racing-mode motivation for those who possess a high degree of fitness. It provides information of effort over 500 metres with average effort per stroke, strokes per minute, distance, energy used and total time.

The action of rowing involves using the big muscle groups: first the legs (which are not locked as you slide back), then the back (which is kept straight and upright), then finally the arms. Rowing vigorously can burn up as many calories as running at 7 mph.

## Ski Machines

By simulating the smooth, dynamic action of cross-country skiing, ski machines can improve aerobic stamina and provide vigorous upper and lower body exercise. This helps to strengthen and tone up legs, thighs, shoulders and arms. Skiing is a low to medium impact exercise that is more suited to the fit and more advanced level exerciser. Ski machines feature sliding footpads and hinged ski poles (levers), or cables running to hand grips which simulate the complete skiing action. They have up to five adjustable resistance levels, in order to exercise both upper and lower body, and an electronic console to monitor time, distance, speed, calorie-burn and pulse. You can, with some designs, even ski uphill!

## Treadmills

Treadmills offer an intensive work-out. They may take the form of motorised or non-motorised machines. They are versatile and, according to design, can vary their speed from a slow or brisk walk to a jog or full sprint. In the latter mode they offer high impact exercise suitable for the intermediate and advanced exerciser. Treadmills should incorporate a non-slip walking/running surface, variable resistance to suit individual body weight and perhaps several incline positions. More expensive models will incorporate a cushion deck to reduce impact. An electronic console can monitor speed, time, distance, calorie-burn and heart rate. Some treadmills offer pre-set work-outs to vary training routines and speed controls can range from 1 to 10 mph. Initially, exercisers may find the feel of the treadmill a little strange. It is similar to the airport travelator, but has more bounce. When ending a training session, gradually slow the machine to a slow walk. Otherwise dizziness can be experienced.

## Steppers or Stairclimbers

Steppers or stairclimbers strengthen the legs, hips, and thighs and have aerobic benefits. They take the form of a stable tubular frame with a safety rail or padded handlebars; independent non-slip pedals attached to hydraulic cylinders that may have six or more variable tension settings to simulate stepping resistance; and an electronic display to provide step count, time, energy consumption and pulse. The action of the stepper imitates the action of steadily walking up stairs, or can be developed into a running motion. Working on air pressure, it is low impact exercise – attained by standing on each step alternately – but imposes little stress on joints. For aerobic benefits, set the machine to low resistance. Muscular endurance can be developed by adjusting to higher resistance which requires a much harder work output.

## Aerobic Riders

These provide all-round exercise. They work on the principle that each rider stroke entails lifting your own body weight. According to design, machines can have a multi-position grip to work arm, back and chest muscles; fully rotational handlebars allowing push or pull training; and second-foot positions allowing high intensity upper body work-out. An electronic console can record repetitions, time and calorie-burn. Some models include adjustable hydraulic resistance with up to 12 settings.

For those interested in toning up muscles there is an extensive range of equipment, from simple devices that target specific body areas such as abdominal trainers, 'bun' trainers that work on thigh and buttock muscles, or exercise training machines previously described (see pages 228ff.). If you are keen to develop strength or muscular endurance, then the use of either free weights (see page 112) or a home gym can be what you want. Home strength equipment may just comprise a bench plus dumb-bells and bar-bells. More advanced modular benches feature attachments for different weight loads and exercises, together with bar-bell stands. Home and multi-gyms are the most versatile.

## Home and Multi-Gyms

Home gyms are designed for use where space permits – perhaps the garage, covered patio or spare room. Multi-gyms are designed for use at sports, health and fitness centres. They demand more space. Both are comprehensive fitness machines that can be used to develop strength or local muscular endurance, dependent on the weights or resistance and repetitions employed. They offer a wide range of exercises and, being fully adjustable, they are easily adapted to meet individual capability. The basic principle of the home or multi-gym is the use of permanently stacked weights that can be load-adjusted to give high or low resistance.

HOW THEY WORK Weights are stacked on a vertical slide within the strong frame of the machine. Cables run vertically from the weights to a pulley, then through other pulleys to a specific exercise bar or feature. On this bar or feature the exerciser will exert muscular effort according to the area of the body where additional strength is required. Once the intended weight to be lifted is selected, a key bolt is inserted in the correct hole in the slide so that only the intended number of stacked weights are lifted. The exerciser then operate the bar or attachment in a slow, controlled manner, raising and

Figure 51: A Home Gym Simplified (showing five examples of exercises possible)

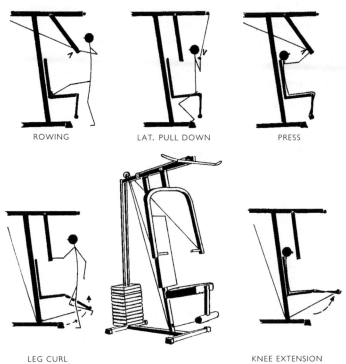

ROWING

LAT. PULL DOWN

PRESS

LEG CURL

KNEE EXTENSION

lowering the load on the slide to the number of reps required. As fitness improves, the key bolt will eventually be removed and inserted in a lower position, so gradually increasing the workload.

The home gym can provide perhaps a 24–30-exercise routine with eight to twelve levels of resistance. The larger multi-gym permits an even wider range of exercises and allows for several people to exercise on the machine at one time, making for maximum utilisation and also ease of supervision. Home and multi-gym training machines make for relatively safe operation with the minimum of practice and supervision. This form of weight training ensures that, should you accidentally misjudge and select too great a load

235

and the drop the weight during an exercise, the weight will fall back on to the stack and not cause injury. Nevertheless, such occurrences should, with a carefully planned programme, be avoidable. Safety of the exerciser should *never* be compromised.

Take note that home and multi-gyms can also be found suitable for the older exerciser, for when they are correctly used less stress is placed on joints than may be experienced with free weights.

## Selecting and Using Exercise Training Machines and Gym Equipment

1. Note the medical precautions and exercise tips on pages 61–4 before considering taking part in any level of physical activity to which you are unaccustomed.

2. Read the manufacturer's instructions so that you understand the purpose of the machine, how it works and any relevant safety rules. Where the use of weights or strong resistance is involved, note the safety points on page 115.

3. Obtain expert advice, then try out equipment under supervision before making a purchase. Initial practice should also be supervised.

4. Before you start exercise sessions, make sure you have a good warm-up, eventually followed by a warm-down. Both should involve flexibility exercises.

5. Never let children near any equipment when it is in use, or be left alone with equipment. Chains, wheels, spokes and weights are potentially dangerous.

# ELEVEN

# Getting Older – Age and Exercise

- The Ageing Process
  - Musculo-Skeletal System
  - Respiratory System
  - Cardiovascular System
  - Lean Body Mass
  - Body Balance
- Dangers of Inactivity
- Slowing Down the Ageing Process
  - Medical Considerations for the Not-so-young
  - Age – Effort Required and Skill Retention
- Retirement
- Exercise – Age Limitations
  - Under 30 Years
  - Between 30 and 45 Years
  - Between 45 and 55 Years
  - Over 55 Years
- For Older People
  - Programme Aims
- Table – Age Recommendations for Competitive Sports, Recreational Games and Activities

Growing to old age as we know it is a relatively new phenomenon. At the beginning of the twentieth century most deaths occurred at about 50 years of age. In but a century our life expectancy has therefore increased by 25 years or more and today some 30 per cent of the UK population is over the age of 65. The period of retirement to be enjoyed by many is now much longer than in the past, but what is important is that our health span matches our life span. Active living is critical to this aim.

Ageing is a condition that affects the whole body and begins from the time of conception. The actual ageing process results from a number of physiological and biochemical reactions that occur within the cells. Not everyone ages at the same rate. Some seemingly grow old before their time, others retain youthful characteristics for many years. Without doubt, genetics play an important part and in some families the qualities of youthfulness are passed on from one generation to another. However, there can be other reasons why certain areas of the world, such as Georgia and Kashmir, have a high population of centenarians. Research into the living habits of these people has revealed two important factors. The first concerns diet: they consume food made up mainly of rice and cereals that are unrefined and have a low calorific value; also their diet contains less fat than diets normally consumed in the Western world. Secondly, they pursue a physically active lifestyle throughout their lives.

In comparison with these active centenarians, it can be said that people who lead inactive lives often seem to register an early deterioration in their physical ability and mental condition. Many people believe that to puff when mildly exerted, become stiff and put on weight are the inevitable legacies of growing older. In fact, these conditions are often the direct result of increasing inactivity and loss of basic fitness. Inactivity, not ageing, is therefore the real enemy of many older people. It can result in them becoming prematurely weaker, fatter, shorter; suffering from ill health, frustration or depression; and being dependent on others.

A sustained programme of moderate exercise combined

with a healthy lifestyle may slow down the ageing process and add years to your life. In a recent scientific study made in Japan, over 200 men between 20 and 85 years old were examined to determine whether those who took exercise regularly were able to remain biologically 'younger' than those who did not exercise. The studies revealed that men who exercise regularly appeared to be between five and seven years biologically 'younger' than the non-exerciser and concluded that regular exercise may increase the life span.

It should be noted that the different components of fitness – strength, speed, suppleness, stamina and skill – do not decline at the same rate. To understand the ageing process we therefore need to look at the body systems affected and to note what happens to them after the age of 35–40.

## Musculo-Skeletal System

Muscle size and strength are normally at their greatest when you are in your 20s. Then, as you grow older, you lose actual muscle mass at an approximate rate of 3–5 per cent every ten years. As the reduction in muscle size and strength occurs, so does the individual's power and speed diminish, because of the reduction in size and number of muscle fibres. Of the components of fitness, strength and speed register the greatest rate of decline with increasing age. This becomes very apparent between 40 and 50 years. By 65 the degree of strength possessed can be 65–70 per cent less than that possessed at 30 years. Some researchers believe that the elderly can lose up to 1.5 per cent of their strength each year.

A loss of strength can give rise to body disorders. Where muscles that serve to control posture become wasted or weak, such as the back and abdominal muscles, low backache and other chronic problems can occur. The muscles that serve the knee, hip and shoulder joints can, through a lack of regular exercise and ageing, become weak. The joints then stiffen, leading to an increased rigidity of connective tissue in joint tendons and ligaments. The loss of lower body strength can, in later life, make walking and climbing stairs difficult and getting up out of a low chair a problem. In one study it was found that 30 per cent of males between 65 and 75 did not have sufficient strength in their thigh muscles to rise easily from a chair; and only half of females over 55 had enough leg strength to climb stairs comfortably. Because of this lack of strength and mobility the heart and lungs are not being exercised and can lose some of their efficiency. Muscles also gradually lose their elasticity and resilience as you grow older. This results in slower reaction time that can, in the extreme, make tasks like driving dangerous.

Ageing causes a decrease in bone density. Bones become weaker due to an overall reduction in bone mass. The reduction in bone density may occur at a rate of 2 per cent per annum. This loss causes increased fragility of the bones (osteoporosis) and an increased tendency to fracture. As already stated, bones need the stimulation of exercise brought about by the pull on tendons and contacting muscles, plus a sustained blood flow to maintain their structural integrity and thickness. A sedentary lifestyle can hasten loss of bone strength and structure, but an active lifestyle makes for bone health and strength.

Suppleness starts to decline from birth as tendons and ligaments thicken during body growth. From as early as the age of 19 the body will lose 1–2 per cent of its flexibility per year. Exercise minimises the stiffening effect and regular suitable suppleness exercises can retain joint flexibility into old age.

## Respiratory System

After the age of about 30 the lungs show a gradual decrease in their elasticity. As the ageing process continues there is a moderate decrease in the strength of the muscles of the chest wall and also the diaphragm, making the lungs lose some of their capacity to expand with each breath inhaled and contact with each breath exhaled. With older people the chest may deepen from front to back, giving a pigeon form, and residual stale air can be left in the lungs; this inefficiency in breathing can tend to foster lung infections such as bronchitis.

The efficiency of the respiratory system is critical to the

maintenance of stamina. Overall, a reduction in stamina appears to occur more slowly than with other components of fitness, though the capacity to utilise oxygen may decline by as much as 20 per cent between the age of 25 and 60.

## Cardiovascular System

After the age of about 35 the heart's ability to pump as much blood as before with each heartbeat decreases slowly at a rate of approximately 5 per cent every ten years. Ageing also affects the blood vessels, for they lose some of their elasticity due to the accumulation of fat and calcium in the artery walls. Arteries cannot then expand to accommodate the flow of blood pumped from the heart and the result is a gradual increase in blood pressure due to resistance of the vessels to the blood flow. After the age of 35 this increase in blood pressure is also registered as approximately 5 per cent every ten years. The major cause of death in the Western world is from disease of the heart and the arterial system that gives rise to strokes and heart attacks. It is believed that regular exercise can reduce these risks. Any exercise programme aiming to prolong life by preventing (or at least delaying) the onset of such cardiovascular disorders must be of the right type, ongoing and, as far as can be judged, at the right intensity.

## Lean Body Mass

The amount of fat-free tissue known as lean body mass diminishes from about the age of 40, mainly due to loss of bone, muscle wastage and a reduction in the size of most organs. The energy-food required to keep the smaller body system functioning effectively decreases with age. However, the same food intake is often maintained, sometimes increased as people get older, resulting in energy being stored as fat. Becoming overweight is therefore not a necessary factor of ageing. All you have to do is look at the build of people in Third World countries where food is short: there is little evidence of older, fat people. What is popularly known as 'middle-age spread' is not caused by middle age, but by too much food and too little exercise taken.

## Body Balance

As we get older the possession of adequate leg strength makes for general mobility around the house and also out of doors, allowing us to do the jobs we want to do and visit the places we enjoy visiting. However, for some people, difficulties in balancing can be a problem in old age and may result in falls and fractures.

Our sense of balance is controlled by the semi-circular fluid-filled canals in the inner ear. The movement of the fluid (endolymph) upon the sense cells in the canals stimulates the cells and gives the brain an appreciation of direction and rate of movement in space. But after recent detailed experiments[1] made by Ian McCloskey, Director of the Prince of Wales Medical Research Institute, Sydney, and his colleague, Richard Fitzpatrick, the conclusion was reached that other balance sensors exist in the calf muscles, contributing to body balance by detecting the lengthening and shortening of the leg muscles as sways occur. McCloskey and Fitzpatrick suspect that the sensors in the calf muscle are the principal sensors when you are standing, while the inner ear sensors take over during rapid movements. As many elderly people suffer from a degenerative condition affecting the nerves (peripheral neuropathy), such a condition in the calves could impair the balance-keeping function of the sensors in the calves and result in a high incidence of falls.

In the light of this research it may be reasonable to assume that any habitual regular exercise of the lower limbs – carried out throughout life and with medical supervision into old age – that develops calf muscle strength, maintains muscle control and stimulates the blood supply to the lower leg muscles and nerves, can only be to our advantage. Some of the exercises that will help develop lower leg strength are heel raising (page 200), foot pushing (page 202), step-ups, stair climbing, cycling, static cycling and walking.

[1] *New Scientist*, 2 November 1996.

The body needs the heart and lungs to be regularly stimulated in order to extract oxygen from the air breathed in and to deliver it together with nutrients to the cells. The more active you are, the less likely you are to be plagued with the degenerative diseases associated with ageing. Modern research has shown that sedentary people have a significantly higher incidence of circulatory and respiratory disease, heart disease, hypertension and strokes, than people who pursue moderate exercise regularly. Studies have also shown that inactive people have a higher incidence of obesity, arthritis, osteoporosis, diabetes and neurological diseases. A lack of exercise when getting older can trigger or exacerbate some of these conditions. Premature ageing can result in depression and early senility.

With the agreement of your doctor, it is never too late to take up some form of exercise, even after years of inactivity. The body will respond to exercise at any time and at any age, provided the exercise is within your personal limits.

SLOWING DOWN THE AGEING PROCESS

Having looked at the effects of ageing on the body and the dangers of inactivity, it is important to examine how to slow down and even, in some instances, reverse the effects of ageing. There follows a summary of the ways in which exercise assists us as we get older.

A programme of regular exercise can dramatically strengthen weak or wasted muscles through the careful use of free weights or weight training machines. Weight bearing exercises such as dancing, running, scout pace and jogging will help prevent bone loss and strengthen weak bones. Exercise sessions do not need to be arduous to be effective. A further recent study was made of the increase in forearm bone strength (density) through the use of tennis balls. Some 100 elderly women were called upon to squeeze a tennis ball for 30 seconds each day. It was found that in six weeks their forearm bone density had increased by over 5 per cent. Physical exercise involving mobility and posture exercises will keep joints mobile, reversing in some cases any increased rigidity and loss of elasticity in tendons and muscles. Such exercise can help counter the possible development of exaggerated spinal curves leading to stooping, a shrinkage in height and the dowager's hump of the female.

Regular exercise keeps the cells of the body infused with adequate amounts of oxygen. With increased age the amount of oxygen distributed to cells starts to decrease and from the mid-twenties inactivity can reduce the cellular activity in body tissue by about 1 per cent each year. Moderate exercise like swimming and cycling improves and maintains the efficiency of the heart and lungs by supplying increased amounts of oxygen to all areas of the body. Perhaps of all types of exercise possible, walking is the safest activity to slow down the ageing of the cardiovascular system. Walking can be pursued throughout a life span. Regular walking can strengthen the heart, make it more efficient, help prevent a rise in blood pressure by keeping the blood vessels pliable and decrease fatty deposits in the arteries – all contributing to preventing heart attacks and strokes.

As stated, while we grow older there is a gradual decline in stamina, though women's stamina declines at a slower rate than men's. Active people maintain their stamina levels for longer than those who lead a sedentary lifestyle. Linked to this area, various studies have been made to compare the cardiovascular systems and breathing capacity of unconditioned people with conditioned people in ages ranging from 40 to 80 years. In one study men between 40 and 60, who had carried out a regular walking programme, were found to have cardiovascular systems twice as efficient as a group of men of similar age who were sedentary. Another study concerned sedentary females and males aged between 60 and 80 who were encouraged to pursue a moderate intensity walking programme for 12 months. At the end of the period the participants registered considerable improvement in their breathing capacity, some as much as 30 per cent. According to the results presented at the 1997 annual conference of the British Association of Sport and Exercise Sciences of a study of elderly people with an average age of 88, the findings concluded that you are never too old to exercise. In the study, held over a period of three months, the elderly participants carried out a twice-weekly programme of circuit training that included walking, chair-rising and stair climbing (preceded by a warm-up and followed by a warm-down). It was found that there were significant improvements in fitness which could bring about an enhanced lifestyle.

Though aerobic activities such as walking, running, cycling and swimming – the 'core activities' – have the most beneficial effect on the heart and lungs, they do not stop the gradual decline in muscle bulk and strength brought on by ageing. This is borne out by comparisons of muscle strength made by Henrik Klitgaard at the August Krogh Institute, Copenhagen, in 1990 between a group of veteran runners and swimmers aged well over 60 – who were, as expected, found to register a high degree of aerobic fitness – and a group of veteran weight trainers in the same age bracket who had trained with fairly heavy weights. Both groups had trained for a decade or more.[1]

Among his findings Klitgaard revealed that not only were the veteran weight trainers stronger than the runners/swimmers, they were in fact stronger than the average man in his late 20s. Further research showed that the veteran runners/swimmers were, as they trained at their prolonged though comparatively low intensity exercise, steadily losing muscle. Klitgaard discovered that the well-defined weight trainers' muscles contained a youthful predominance of well-developed fast twitch fibres – giving instant strength and making for explosive movements – whereas many of the fast twitch fibres of the runner/swimmer group had withered away.

There was therefore the possibility that, as the runner/swimmer group grew older into their 80s or 90s, the difficulties and dangers associated with lack of body strength (for example, rising from a chair or experiencing a tendency to fall) would be as great as their peers who, over the years, had done little or no exercise. On the other hand the possession and retention of muscle bulk, incorporating many fast twitch fibres – as displayed by the weight trainers – made for the explosive movement which underpins one's capability to move out of the way of traffic, heave that suitcase on to the

[1] *Reader's Digest*, April 1997.

rack, or do moderately hard jobs around the house safely. These of course are all factors that contribute to personal mobility and quality of life as we grow older.

General weight training with fairly heavy weights, carried out with expert supervision in middle age and continued as a pattern of life (with necessary reductions in weights as age increases), can therefore have considerable benefits. These benefits are greatly enhanced when weight training is combined with any of the core aerobic exercises that can improve endurance, reduce blood pressure and decrease the risk of heart disease and heart attacks. Consequently a sound degree of general fitness can be achieved.

A personal cross-training programme incorporating aerobic and strengthening exercises, carefully compiled and modified in intensity to meet the requirements of the older person, is a good way to mould the two elements. At the same time, it produces a balanced, interesting exercise schedule. The aerobic element could be selected, according to age and ability, from the indoor stationary activities of walking, running, scout pace or cycling; or from any of these activities performed out of doors, including free cycling. Take note, however, of the considerations outlined on pages 248ff. regarding limitations.

The weight training aspects should also be adapted in intensity and could include a dumb-bell or bar-bell circuit or an exercise circuit using body weight, or a combination of such exercises. Isometric exercises could also be included provided they are those that do not pose problems for older people by greatly raising blood pressure.


## Medical Considerations for the Not-so-young

The importance of being checked out by your physician before you undertake any level of physical activity to which you are unaccustomed cannot be too greatly emphasised for those over 40 and particularly those of a greater age. Under no circumstances should the elderly be exposed to exercises or activities that are exhaustive or stressful. They should always exercise within their limits and never struggle to do more than is reasonably possible (see also page 61, Medical Precautions).

As previously stressed, it is never too late to get fit and to keep fit, though a 50-year-old may take twice as long as a 30-year-old to reach the same standard if both were to start from the same level of fitness. The former's progressions will also need to be more gentle; but it is often found that the 50-year-old, having more determination and fewer distractions, is more likely to succeed in his quest for fitness. There is no doubt that as you get older a more deliberate effort is required to maintain a good level of fitness. For example, though it is possible for a rugby football player in his mid-30s to play as well as he did in his 20s, he has to train much harder than he did when younger to retain that ability.

The skills and techniques we have picked up over the years can serve as a buffer against the ageing process, though there can be considerable variations between the rate of decline of different skills. This depends on how much physical effort is required to carry out the skill and also whether it is 'self-paced' (in which the movement is initiated by the performer) or is carried out in an 'open' situation (where the movement is a response to actions initiated by an opponent). In the first instance a well-motivated, mature and fit archer, rifle shot, golfer, skier or dancer may retain much of his/her skills level despite the passing years. In open situations – where physical effort perhaps requires pace, power and acceleration as demanded in a rugby centre's intended side-step; or the particular response required to return the volley from a squash opponent – the level of quick reaction and effort needed to succeed may be beyond the average older player's capabilities.

## RETIREMENT

Retirement is the time to relax without the stresses and strains imposed by work, but it is a mistake to take things too easily. Your aim should be to make yourself fitter than you were before retiring – you have a wonderful opportunity, for the time is there to spend profitably, perhaps through regular enjoyable golf sessions, long rambles or cycle tours. Keeping fit does not mean you have to be wildly energetic. It means being physically active within your own limits, so that the body is ticking over nicely, the joints are being well used, body strength is kept up and the brain remains stimulated with that feeling of well-being. Activities such as bowling and ballroom dancing will also keep you supple and in good shape. They also have important social values. Gardening can be another way of getting exercise. Digging and hedge cutting help maintain strength and balance; weeding keeps the joints flexible.

Aerobic activities such as moderate cycling, walking and swimming are ideal. They assist in weight control, keep the heart and lungs in good order and help to keep the legs strong so that you can get around with minimum effort. In most instances, it is best for the older person to avoid jogging and running, as they can induce back and joint trouble. Competitive sports can also be too demanding, but sports such as skiing, canoeing and sailing can continue to be enjoyed, as can many other recreational pursuits and dance activities. Figure 52 gives, in broad terms, a suggested guide to the age range suited for different sports and activities. It can be seen that the scope for all ages is vast, offering wide exercise opportunities.

## EXERCISE — AGE LIMITATIONS

Research workers have concluded that habitual physical activity, particularly of an aerobic nature, can help maintain organic vigour, a youthful physique and general flexibility, and also delay the onset of degenerative conditions associated with ageing. Often people continue to enjoy participating in competitive sport, despite their advancing years, because they have maintained a regular training programme. Though the training effect registered can be highest when we are young, with the accompanying peak performance normally achieved during that relatively short period of our lives, the habitual repetition of suitable physical activity over the whole span of life is of far greater importance.

Examples can be found where older individuals who,

having regularly participated in competitive sport, and being both physically and medically very fit, have recorded some remarkable achievements. Billy Meredith obtained his international football cap for Wales at the age of 45. Sir Stanley Matthews was still playing English First Division football at the age of 50 and continued to play in English divisional football for many years Perhaps one of the most remarkable achievements of an older athlete was that of Dimitrion Yordanidis, who ran the marathon in Greece. He was 98 years old and recorded a time of 7 hours, 33 minutes.

These athletes are exceptions. For those who have *not* exercised regularly, it is wise to observe certain age limitations. The activities selected should relate to the body-type of person (see page 49). For example, a heavy fat-prone person (endomorph) would benefit from activity that is weight-supporting such as cycling or swimming. On the other hand, a lightly built person (ectomorph) may be well suited to walking and running. Take note that whatever your age, if you have any reason to doubt your medical condition get yourself checked out by your doctor *before* undertaking a level of physical activity to which you are unaccustomed. The recommendations outlined below are for those who have not exercised regularly, but they are not meant to be prescriptive.

## Under 30 Years

Provided you do not have some obvious medical problem, you should be able to embark on any beginner's progressive exercise programme based on one or more of the core activities of walking, running, cycling or swimming. After attaining a sound standard of fitness, should you wish to participate in any game that is potentially demanding – such as squash – then your introduction to the game should be controlled in both intensity and duration so as not to overtax the body.

### Between 30 and 45 Years

If you are under 40, in good health and with no medical problems, you should be able to enjoy participating in any of the core activities but with more gentle progressions. However, if you are over 40 or are planning some strenuous exercise, get your doctor's approval before you start. Take care to ensure that the intensity of your participation is initially moderate and then gradually increased, but never allow yourself to be put under great stress or to become exhausted.

### Between 45 and 55 Years

First of all, get a check-up with your doctor. Start with a progressive walking programme and only after some time, when you are really walking fit, should you consider taking part in more intense exercise. Those under 50 may wish to progress to light jogging or running, but note that the older person may find jogging can result in stress and strain of the back ligaments, discs and verebrae. Jogging and running, particuarly on hard surfaces, can give knee problems and hip and foot injuries. Alternate walking with short periods of either gentle jogging/running/striding can help to avoid these problems and will build up aerobic fitness.

You may wish to progress to a racket game. As far as casual individual recreational games are concerned (as distinct from individual competitive games with a high stress level), the under-50s will find badminton a less demanding game than squash. Squash is a game that many believe to be best reserved for the fit younger person and not those approaching middle age, though there are many successful older but experienced competitive players. As far as recreational games are concerned, volleyball, being less taxing than basketball, is more suitable for under-50s. Many people in the 45–55 age group find that the less arduous exercises of brisk walking, golf, cycling, static cycling and swimming meet all their exercise needs.

Over 55 Years

Before you start exercising, get a check-up with your doctor. Again, start with a progressive walking programme. Swimming, golf, cycling and stationary cycling are also good forms of exercise, but progressions should be gentle. Avoid more vigorous activities such as competitive games, jogging and running.

## FOR OLDER PEOPLE

With advancing years, into the 70s and 80s, the preventative effects of moderate but regular physical exercise, along with a suitable diet, enough rest and sleep, plus adequate medical and dental care, are of considerable importance. The control of body weight, release of tension and emotional stress, maintenance of bodily functions are also relevant in the quest for and retention of health and fitness. Many people in their 70s and 80s are very fit and healthy because they have always been very active. But for those who do not enjoy such a standard of fitness, with medical approval, every encouragement should be given to doing some exercise and keeping mobile. Strength and suppleness exercises are important for older people, though care must be taken not to strain or overload joints. Strength-developing machines like the multi-gym are suitable: less stress is placed on joints than when using conventional weights, but their use *must* be closely supervised.

Those elderly people who cannot bring themselves to take part in regular exercise of some form can be at risk from bone-related disorders and loss of mobility. If they are up to it, they should be encouraged to get out of the house every day and take a ten-minute stroll. Those who can should be encouraged to walk a little further each day, provided it does not overtax them. The exercise will make them more alert and fresh, help to keep the digestive system working properly and also boost morale. What is important is that the elderly always exercise within their limits.

## Programme Aims

Those of advancing years should ideally have a personal programme, however modest, to meet their needs and be incorporated into their way of life. Thus they will maintain their physical potential and achieve a satisfying self-image. This programme should aim to help them:

a. Maintain their energy and vitality by enjoying physical activities suited to their ability.
b. Maintain their interest in life and their surroundings.
c. Preserve their mental capacity.
d. Keep up a good appearance.
e. Have a balanced relationship with others.
f. Where possible, obtain protection from chronic degenerative conditions.
g. Allow them to live without being greatly dependent on others.

It is important for the elderly always to have something to look forward to: an interest to fill their life, perhaps a hobby or specific project that stimulates and serves as a challenge – for example, taking a language course, learning to swim or, for some, walking to the library. It is all part of being active, and activity makes for good health in mind and body.

Figure 52: Age Recommendations for Participation in Competitive Sports, Recreational Games and Activities

As you grow older, all exercise should be of a less strenuous nature. The following tables give broad age ranges which are suggestions and not meant to be in any way prescriptive. The age recommendations for competitive sports relate to serious competitive involvement and assume that participation takes place only after full physical and mental preparation has been undertaken to meet the demands of play. The age recom- mendations for recreational games and activities assume that participants are adequately prepared – both in fitness and technique – but that a less demanding

## Competitive Sports

| SPORTS | AGE RECOMMENDATION UNDER | SPORTS | AGE RECOMMENDATION UNDER |
|---|---|---|---|
| Athletics | 40 | Orienteering | 40 |
| Badminton | 50 | Riding | 50 |
| Basketball | 40 | Rowing | 40 |
| Canoeing | 40 | Rugby | 40 |
| Long distance | | Skating | 40 |
| Slalom | | Speed | |
| Sprint | | Skiing | 40 |
| Cricket | 50 | Downhill | |
| Cycle racing | 40 | Langlauf | |
| Endurance running | 40 | Soccer | 40 |
| Fencing | 40 | Squash | 40 |
| Golf | 50 | Swimming | 40 |
| Gymnastics | 35 | Table tennis | 40 |
| Handball | 40 | Tennis | 50 |
| Hockey | 40 | Trampolining | 35 |
| Judo | 40 | Volleyball | 40 |
| Motorcycle | 35 | Water skiing | 40 |
| Cross-country Trials | | Water polo | 35 |

## Recreational Games and Activities

| GAMES AND ACTIVITIES | AGE RECOMMENDATION | GAMES AND ACTIVITIES | AGE RECOMMENDATION |
|---|---|---|---|
| Archery | All Ages | Motoring | All Ages |
| Bowling | | Riding | |
| Indoor | | Sailing | |
| Lawn | | Casual | |
| Camping | | Shooting | |
| Canoe touring | | Clay | |
| Croquet | | Pistol | |
| Cycling | | Rifle | |
| Dancing | | Rough | |
| Darts | | Skating | |
| Fishing | | Casual | |
| Coarse | | Swimming | |
| Fly | | Walking | |
| Sea | | Weight training | |
| Gardening | | Yoga | |
| Golf | | | |

and more relaxed approach is made, allowing the involvement of a wider age span with activities carried out at the pace of the individual.

Note: if you have any reason to doubt your medical condition, consult your doctor *before* undertaking a level of physical activity to which you are unaccustomed.

# Further Reading

Bowerman, J., & Harris, W.E., *Jogging* (Corgi, 1968)
Cooper, K.H., *Aerobics* (Bantam, 1968)
                     *The New Aerobics* (Bantam, 1975)
Davies, M.B., *Physical Training Games and Athletics in Schools* (Allen & Unwin, 1951)
Egger, G., Champion, N., & Hurst, G., *The Fitness Leader's Exercise Bible* (Kangaroo Press, 1996)
Fairney A., & Wilson, J., *Osteoporosis – Booklet for Patients* (St Mary's NHS Trust Hospital, London)
Gargrave, R., *Step Exercises* (Boatswain Press, 1993)
Goodsell, A., *Your Personal Trainer* (Boxtree, 1994)
Hardy, R., *The Longbow* (Patrick Stevens, 1976)
Hazeldine, R., *Fitness for Sport* (Crowood Press, 1985)
Health Education Authority, *Getting Active, Feeling Fit Exercise: Why Bother?*
Jackson, G., *Fitness and Exercise* (Salamander, 1985)
Jarvis, M.A., *Swimming for Teachers and Youth Leaders* (Faber & Faber, 1947)
Katz, J., *Fitness Works* (Leisure Press, 1988)
Larson, L.A., & Michelman, H., *International Guide to Fitness and Health* (Crown Publications, 1973)
National Osteoporosis Society, *Exercise and Physiotherapy in the Prevention and Treatment of Osteoporosis* (1995)
Office of Health Economics, Osteoporosis (1990)
Ripley, A. & Ferris, L., *Forty Plus* (Stanley Paul, 1992)
Rosser, M.O., *Body Fitness* (Hodder & Stoughton, 1995)
Royal Air Force, *RAF Physical Fitness Handbook* (1961)
Schubert, J., *Cycling for Fitness* (Oxford Illustrated Press, 1989)
Sharp, C., *Fitness for Life* (Piatkus, 1996)
Snowdon, L., & Humphreys, M., *Fitness Walking* (Mainstream, 1992)
Williams, P.F., *Canoe Skills and Canoe Expedition Techniques for Teachers and Leaders* (Pelham, 1967)
                     *Hill Walking* (Pelham, 1979)